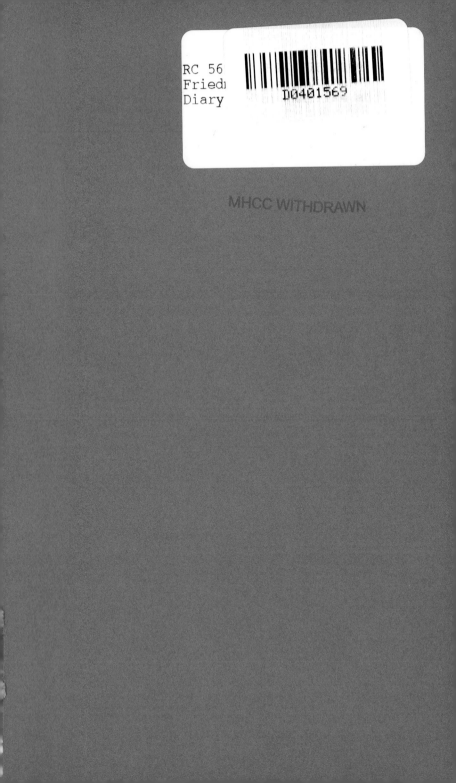

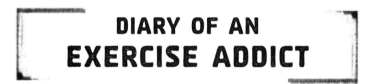

# DIARY OF AN
# EXERCISE ADDICT

*A memoir by Peach Friedman*

## gpp
### life

Guilford, Connecticut
An imprint of The Globe Pequot Press

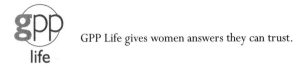

GPP Life gives women answers they can trust.

GPP Life is an imprint of The Globe Pequot Press.

Text design by Sheryl P. Kober

Library of Congress Cataloging-in-Publication Data
Friedman, Peach.
  Diary of an exercise addict : a memoir / by Peach Friedman.
    p. cm.
  ISBN-13: 978-0-7627-4896-9
  1.  Friedman, Peach—Mental health.  2.  Exercise addiction—Patients—United States—Biography.  I. Title.
  RC569.5.E94F75 2009
  616.85'260092—dc22
  [B]
                                          2008017254

Printed in the United States of America

10 9 8 7 6 5 4 3 2 1

*This book is for my mother and father.*

## A Note to The Reader

*Exercise bulimia is a newly recognized eating disorder. It is identified by a compulsion to purge calories through excessive exercise. I refer in my book to exercise addiction and compulsive exercise, which I use as interchangeable phrases for exercise bulimia.*

# Prologue

*On a recent Saturday evening, Jeffrey and I hurried to get ready for a dinner party. I tried on the same three dresses several times: one was too dressy, he thought, and I didn't like the way it shaped my arms. One was a little slutty, I thought, and he agreed—too short, too much skin. And the third was too summery. It's late fall; dressing for the seasons is somewhat confusing in a Northern California climate. Today, for instance, it's eighty degrees, but there are pumpkins on doorsteps and Starbucks is advertising its spicy latte. I wound up choosing the dressier dress that didn't flatter my arms, forgot to put on perfume, and off we drove.*

*Nice people, all of them. Genuine, friendly, down to earth. I sat with two women I hadn't met before, sipping wine and talking about working out, about exercise: a common conversation among ladies. With my back to Jeffrey, I wondered if he was listening—silently I hoped he was overhearing this conversation. He's learned a lot since we've been together, about eating disorders and exercise compulsions. He's learned a lot about what I deem healthy behavior and what concerns me. It was too noisy for me to tell if he was leaning forward, listening to us, or if he had engaged in some other conversation behind me, but it quickly didn't matter, because I was wrapped up with my two new friends.*

*They were discussing the pros and cons of their gym in Sacramento, so I told them that I'm a personal trainer, and that I educate about eating disorders and the risks of exercise addictions. One of the women laughed,* Oh, I wish I had that problem! *I could see the other woman scan my body, check out my size. I thought to myself,* I wish I'd worn the other dress. . . .

Boulder is beautiful in autumn: the sky pure blue, cloudless and bright, the air fresh with changing seasons and falling leaves. Up in the mountains above Boulder the aspen trees are turning. I like driving up the canyon to this huge rock situated off the road somewhere between the small mountain towns of Nederland and Ward. When I lived here with my boyfriend Christopher, we would pack a picnic lunch and sit there, on the rock, gazing at the landscape in the crisp, sunny air. I'm beautiful this fall, too. It's my senior year of college, and my flesh is slightly carved away, my hair straighter than usual, the hem of it flat, solid, even, the whole combination of which gives me a look of impermeability.

(It was, in fact, such an impossibly temporary phase. Nothing lasted that year, or in the years to follow. About my hair I later wondered, was it the Boulder temperature that steadied the fall of my locks? Was it the weather, the dryness, my diet? I lost so many long white strands down the shower drain that fall and kept calling home to ask, *Am I eating enough chicken? Is there a pollutant in the water?*)

My mother is visiting. I pick her up at the airport in Denver. I look dazzling, with deep blue-black eyelashes and those flat blonde tresses swooping my shoulder blades in the back. I'm wearing some unusually chic yet Boulderesque combination of clothes: a V-neck whooshed in a swirl of colors, a knee-length straight and stretchy black skirt, and fuchsia platform thong sandals. Mom always manages to outdo me, her diamond earrings thrice the rocks of what feel like chips in my own lobes. And on this trip, despite my mother's grief—pain I don't yet know about—she steps off the airplane in straight suede pants and an olive leather jacket. She looks Parisian, tiny and sophisticated.

# OCTOBER 21, 2000

It's another gorgeous, sunny afternoon in Colorado, and my mother and I are sitting together outside the Boulder Tea House eating its famous hummus on our salads, sipping at our soy chais. I've just said I would move to Boston and marry a Harvard man. That perfect autumn blend of sun and breeze is on my back, warming my skin through my T-shirt. The leaves in the park across the street are falling, crisp yellows and oranges, and all around us college students, mothers with strollers, businessmen, and joggers look like they're almost prancing in the sunlight. Boulder is unsurpassable in autumn: that ideal combination of cool in the mornings and warm all afternoon, with such a bright sky it makes you want to sun your legs. Or maybe it's only so perfect through my polished approach to life this month. Everything is perfect. Everything is just fine. I am stronger than ever. I tell myself again, *I am stronger than ever.*

I tell Mom we should get our nails done. I tell her that I need to get to the gym before dinner. I tell her that I need to market myself for marriage. Mom says, *I'm here to tell you everything will be okay, darling girl. I'm taking a bit of a break from family life.* She's squeezing my hand now, our faces close together, and I'm noticing a chicken pox scar on her cheek, near her lips and nose. She says, *I've rented an apartment, just to get to be a girl! What do you think of that? We'll still have Christmas at home and then I'll spend a few months on my own. It's a darling apartment, all white, and we'll bring in white orchids and a big mirror, that one we both liked from the catalog. Not to worry, my darling girl, there is nothing to worry about.*

It's as if one more brick slides out of place in that moment. Life as I know it is already crumbling: My boyfriend Christopher and I have just broken up. College will soon be over, and I have yet to consider work, a career. I am clinging to flat, smooth hair and daily runs for solace.

*Everything is just fine,* I tell myself again.

Now, sitting up straight, declaring my pursuits to my mother, always looking outside myself for answers (the Harvard husband, the trip to the gym), she manages to tell me in a single sentence that she's leaving my father but *everything is fine.*

And everything is fine, because I'm numb. I nod, *Of course, I understand.* And I do—I have watched my parents fight through my childhood and teenage years. I feel surprisingly calm, despite the wreckage that's mounting in my body.

Often, when a person is emotionally overwhelmed, when a person is flooded with emotion, they find a way to disconnect, to skip the pain altogether. I am a fast learner.

In bed that night, I eat the cookies we bought that afternoon to help us feel safe in the bed-and-breakfast where we are sharing a room for the weekend.

I don't think I need cookies to feel safe, but I know my mother does. I followed her around the grocery store *Oh yes*ing her, watching her move—her hair, the lines of her arms, the purse in her lips, deciding, choosing, selecting so delicately what she would let herself eat, what was good enough, fine enough, perfect. I packed a weekend bag to take with me to the B&B, so we could curl up together until Sunday, watching videos at night and talking, cuddling, snacking. When I was growing up, Mom always kept food by her bed at night, laid out on a napkin. Usually peanut butter on bread, or a banana.

Sometimes she had one bite, sometimes two, but most evenings it lay there beside her, an altar to resistance, to discipline, to keeping away, until morning, when it was stale and she'd wrap the napkin around the piece of bread with peanut butter, the cookie, the banana, and drop it in the kitchen trash. I didn't understand how this distance of food from mouth could keep my mother feeling safe, not yet I didn't. Three or four chocolate cookies are down past my throat soon enough, and soon enough it feels wrong to have them there.

I learn later that Mom didn't keep uneaten food at her bedside to feel safe in staying away; rather, she kept the food there to know it was readily available in case she got hungry. It was there if she needed it, like an extra blanket just in case the heat didn't work. After a decade of starving herself, the thought of sleeping in a strange place without a safety snack close by was unsettling. But I don't know her that well yet, and I don't understand that not eating can be used for many things. I am just starting to learn what it means to be a beautiful woman, a woman like my mother, and I have decided it means not eating cookies that are set up perfectly on a napkin. It means pursing your lips and choosing selectively. It means the world will be okay, no matter what, no matter if you are leaving your husband but can't say it.

## EARLY OCTOBER 2000

It's two weeks before my mom's trip to Colorado. In a one-tint-warmer Boulder shade of autumn, I'm flying east to Boston to see my boyfriend Christopher, under the guise of visiting my brother Nat and scoping the city for a potential post-college move. Christopher is at school in Connecticut; he's getting a ride with a friend to meet me in Boston for the weekend. Last year we lived together in Colorado. Christopher took a semester off school to work as a research assistant for a professor at CU. He spent his days skiing up into the mountains to collect water samples while I took walks in the sunshine and studied poetry at Naropa, the small Buddhist liberal arts college where I am working toward my BA.

~~~

Christopher and I met in high school, through friends. I remember the first night we saw each other: It was my eighteenth birthday, a Saturday night in June, and I went to a concert at the small nightclub in our hometown of Charlottesville, Virginia, down by the railroad tracks with a couple of girlfriends. Bruce Hornsby made a surprise appearance that night, and everyone cheered and stayed late. I was wearing a long, blue wraparound hippie skirt with a thin, spaghetti-strap undershirt top, Birkenstock sandals, and a ribbon in my hair. Christopher was behind me with his brother, talking to my girlfriends, who he knew from middle school. They introduced us. His smile was enormous, light and happy. We ran into each other again in the fall, early during our senior year of high school, on the downtown mall, where all the youth of Charlottesville still collect on Friday nights. Usually there's a band playing. Always there's flirting and smoking and dancing. Christopher and I fell in love. I couldn't resist his sweet, happy approach to life, his steadiness, and his bright, flashing eyes.

Like most young couples, we had to make decisions when we went off to college. I spent a mixed-up year at a small school in North Carolina before transferring to Naropa in Boulder. Christopher went to Wesleyan, in Connecticut. We collected frequent flier miles and spent long, whispering nights together over holidays at home in Virginia. And when I moved to Colorado, Christopher said he would come with me. But it wasn't until our junior year when he finally took a semester off to live in Boulder. And after that, he took off again to study abroad in Africa. I was heartbroken. I remember we were driving through some mountain town in Colorado when he told me he'd decided to apply for the program. He said, *I looked at all the options, and this one scared me the most. That's why I want to do it.*

We wrote letters obsessively. Okay, I wrote letters obsessively. I have them still saved on my computer: I typed them all, at least one a day, often more, and mailed them to Tanzania. He wrote as best he could, sweet love notes, and once or twice sent photographs. It was during this semester that I began to tweak the way I ate, and how often I exercised. I was so lonely, and so anxious. If too much time passed without a letter, I would panic. I mapped out our life in those months. I wrote him letters with detailed plans for how we'd spend the summer when he returned. And I worked with a therapist who suggested, perhaps, that regular exercise might help ease my stress and anxiety. So I joined the local YMCA and started jogging. And lo and behold, I found that I felt better after a hard run. I also discovered that it changed my body. And people noticed. I wrote Christopher letters about my newfound interest in exercise. I told him, *I've lost a bit of weight, you may notice.* He wrote back and said, *Whatever you do, don't lose your butt!* When he stepped off the airplane in June, the first thing he said to me was, *Peachie, you look thin.*

Now, I was certainly thinner than before, but I wasn't, at this point, skinny or sick or starved. I have never been heavy or overweight. I have always been in the normal range for my height, and never before had I tried to lose or gain weight. I didn't even try to lose weight that semester: I tried only to find solace from my heartache. But I learned one method of coping, and I became attached to that method, and to what it yielded: a slightly leaner and more toned body. A body that gleaned more interest from men, more envy from women. I stuck with it and paid attention to what I ate, too. Instead of eating what I craved, I drilled my mother, asking her what was healthy, what was good for me, what would help me keep this nice lean body.

When Christopher returned from Africa, I enrolled in Naropa's Summer Writing Program and he found a job in Crested Butte, a six-hour drive away, and a drive I grew to love, slowly winding my way up and over Cottonwood Pass, beginning to feel that the landscape of the Rocky Mountains was mine to keep.

We spent our last weeks of that same summer on a drive together, from Colorado through Utah and Idaho, and into Portland, Oregon, where we visited my uncle and his family. Then we headed through Eugene to the coast and spent the most romantic vacation of my life to date traveling together, in my small pickup truck, down Highway 1, and eventually into San Francisco. Most of those afternoons we napped lazily in the bed of my truck, the tailgate open and cool Pacific breezes soothing us. We walked on the beaches at sunset, hooded sweatshirts keeping us warm. We took photographs in the Redwoods and made love tucked in wet, wooded campgrounds. Christopher would drive while I stretched my legs out the window and wrote in my journal.

~~~

This fall Christopher is back at Wesleyan, and I've moved into a big house on the hill in Boulder, with a bunch of CU girls and a new look. Christopher and I are used to being at a distance, physically. But now, with real life looming on the post-college horizon, I'm nervous as I pack my bags for Boston.

I'm wearing those same fuchsia platform thong sandals on the airplane that I will wear to pick up my mother at the airport in Denver later in the month. I wear the same deep and heavy mascara, the same diamond earrings, the same skirt. The first night of my long-weekend trip I spend alone with my brother Nat, eating prawns at Legal Seafood in Cambridge, the one near MIT, and having the first honest conversation we've had in years. We are on the brink, Nat and I, of friendship. He has finished school, is launching a software company, wears beautiful, tailored clothes, and has maids polishing the hardwood floors of his apartment. We talk about our parents, about what it was like growing up, about how we're changing as adults, and what we believe in. Nat is passionate and I look up to him.

In the morning I go for a run on the paths near his house, my consistently flat blonde hair, like a gift from a celebrity magazine, brushing my shoulder blades in perfect ponytail form as I jog and think about Christopher. In the afternoon, with Nat at work, I sit at his open dining room table, with the semicircular windows looking out over Beacon Street, listening to the thrashing of the C-line train below. Boston is colder than Boulder in October. The sunlight is less yellow, the sky less blue. But on the East Coast again, in the Northeast now, I feel a tickle of excitement in my guts and groin: what it might mean to be a Bostonian, to live this life. How my wardrobe might be different. More black. How my days might be different. More coffee. Toying with the idea of moving here after graduation, I am supposed to be investigating the city to see if I can fit right in, but instead I am pacing my brother's living room, tromping over his Oriental carpets in those same fuchsia sandals, waiting for Christopher to ring the doorbell, to call. I am checking my hair and eyelashes in the mirror over the piano. I am thinner than when we met, Christopher and I. I am more beautiful, obsessed with my beauty.

Which, as it turns out, is in the eye of the beholder. Sweet Christopher eventually clops up the steps to Nat's brownstone and takes me in in one breath, one fleeting eye-dance of can't quite land anywhere on my body, and blurts, *Your eyes look funny.*

We go out that night, with Nat and his friends, to Charlie's Kitchen in Harvard Square. (I would later spend countless nights scarfing burgers and fries, doing shots, chugging beers, smoking cigarettes there with Nat and his friends, but then, that first time, I didn't know to remember the place: to drink in not just the Hoegaarden, but the mirrored walls, the jukebox, the face of each individual waitress—the waitresses in black and studded belts who worked for years at Charlie's, who got hit on and went home with several of my brother's friends, my brother himself.) I sit across from Christopher, the mix of music and booze and the chill of autumn flushing our skin, pulsing out my triceps and the tops of my feet. He isn't used to my designer jeans, my smooth, flat hair. We aren't used to being twenty-one and drunk together, but here we are. I look at his wide smile across the table and ask when he thinks we should get married.

It's not so out of the blue. We've talked about this before. We've even imagined where we'd hold the ceremony. *I dunno,* he says, *how about when we're like, twenty-three? Yeah,* I say, *that sounds about right. Cause I want to have kids when I'm like, twenty-six, so that'll give us a few years. And twenty-two . . . that's just too young. Yeah, twenty-three will be good,* he says. After the drive home, back across the bridge, back to Beacon Street in Nat's shiny BMW, blasting Radiohead and that unshakeable feeling that life will never change, that it should always be this good, this free, this surrounded with beauty and men and love, Christopher and I fuck on the air mattress in Nat's living room. It's only the second time I can remember ever fucking Christopher: *fucking* like we really had something to lose, something to hold onto, something to possess and dominate.

We break up within days of my return to Boulder, sniffling on the phone, talking in metaphors of letting birds go, and whispering thank yous across the wires. It's my initiative: There is some new divide between us, I can feel it, and though we love each other enormously, I believe that if we continue trying to make it work, we will be forcing something. I had already bought a ticket to fly to Connecticut one weekend in early November. Christopher wants me to still use it. *It's okay, Peachie, you can come out anyway. We can just hang out.* But I'm trying hard to move on. I tell him no. I go to bars with my new girlfriends, let men hit on me, enjoying the power I have with my designer clothes and perfect hair. I also have a huge crush on a guy in my program at school.

Everyone asks me why I ended it with Christopher. *It was just time,* I tell people. *Nothing bad happened. We didn't have a fight and we don't hate each other. It's just that I want to end it now, before it does get ugly. I want to always cherish this as my first love. Christopher has been my best friend, but it's time for us both to try something new, to grow up.*

Still, we make an agreement that even though we're breaking up, we will not fully close the door until one of us says it's closed for good.

## CHRISTMAS 2000

I, as it turns out, hold onto that hope more than he does. We talk on the phone often between our breakup and the winter holiday. Christopher even invites me to spend a weekend with his friends in the mountains. But suddenly there is a break in the phone calls, and when we talk again Christopher un-invites me and says he has a new girlfriend. I don't blame him. We are not together anymore. He is right to move on. I have been dating in Boulder, a fellow poet named Jack who let me put my head in his lap while my roommate drove us from bar to bar, my feet dangling out the window, skirt falling around my waist. But it isn't serious. My mind is on other pursuits. By Christmas I am already down a few pounds, my hair miraculously even straighter and blonder, my clothes more expensive with every wear. My departure from the young earthy love Christopher and I shared has come in the form of a calloused growing up, but also a delicate, inevitable return to my roots.

Christopher knocks on the door of my parents' big house one morning with a Christmas present for me. It's a CD, and he asks me why I don't have a present for him. I don't know how to respond; I want to say, *Duh! Because we broke up, because you have a new girlfriend, maybe?* but I don't say that. Instead, I ask if he wants to come with me to feed the dogs I'm watching over while a friend of the family vacations out of town. When we get to the house, Christopher tries to hold me, or kiss me, and I push him away, back against the sink, the cowl-neck of my red sweater just in the periphery of my eyesight. *Christopher, you can't do that, you're with someone else.* He says he isn't sure it's for real, he says the love hasn't left him, the love for me, he says,

*How can we not hang out, how can I not hold your hand, touch your hair?* I'm confused. I'm heartbroken. He has a girlfriend, so why is he trying to hold my hand? I know why: He loves me and I love him, too, and we both agree that it was time to move on but suddenly, being here, side by side, so soon, we don't know how to behave. I want to kiss him but I don't want to feel any pain or longing.

It's cold outside and the dog's water is frozen. We force sharp shards of ice from the plastic bucket, refill it with warm water; I'll be back later in the day to check on it.

Christopher won't, though, and I will see him only once more before late spring, by which time I'll have truly transformed, truly shrunk, and will be unrecognizable in only skin and bones, my twelve-year-old sister's clothes hanging from my hard, chipping form, my lips purple, and my hair no longer shining. Still, even then, he will knock on the door of my parents' big house and, as we walk away together, reach for my hand.

As it happens, I return to Boulder for only one night in January, to pack up my pickup truck and bring my belongings back home, back to my breaking family in Virginia, where I feel I need to be, but where I declare I am returning in order to help my adolescent sister find some stability during our parents' separation.

# EARLY JANUARY 2001

Dad flies with me one morning out of Charlottesville, through D.C., and into Denver. In the airport that morning we see Christopher's oldest brother waiting for his flight out, back to Chicago, where he's in chiropractic school. He overhears me tell Dad that my knee hurts and leans back across the chairs to suggest a strengthening exercise. I'm happy to see him, for him to see me looking lovely and lean, but I resent his advice. When the small propeller plane takes off for D.C., Dad and I giggle over the noise of the engines.

From Denver we take a bus to Boulder, like I always did returning to school, though this time is different. It's my last time, and with my father now, how strange. Within two hours we have everything I could possibly want to keep shoved in the bed of my small, lightweight pickup. I say good-bye to no one and start the three-day drive back across Kansas, Missouri, and Kentucky, into the night of winter with my father, aiming for home. Each of those three mornings I wake up before sunrise to run on the treadmill in the slightly varying hotel gyms. Then we grab snacks for the day and head out together across the widest stretch of our country.

Later, Daddy will remember the drive fondly. But the discomfort in my own skin is increasing, and though the confusion between my parents is not my particular issue, I feel awkward on this long road trip: just me and Dad, with so much pain lurking in the space between us. Daddy and I butt heads— we are stubborn, strong-willed, and opinionated people, both of us. I got those qualities from him, and I love them in myself, but I hate the same traits in him when we have to resolve any kind of situation. Right now we aren't hurting because of our father-daughter relationship; we're hurting because we've both lost love. Another father-daughter pair might use this as an opportunity to feel close to each other, but in our case I feel the space between us only widen.

I stuck my finger down my throat once or twice last week at home, hoping for I'm not sure what, because I couldn't quite get the undigested food to come back up. Mom has talked with me a bit about their separation. Daddy really only says that it wasn't his idea and he's not happy about it. I don't know what happened, but I'm convinced something *happened,* though Mom swears that isn't the case. Maybe, I think, it's like me and Christopher— maybe it's just time? But I'm not convinced of this, and I feel like a little kid who isn't being told the whole story.

All I know for sure is that something isn't right: not with me, or with my parents, and living my last semester of college in Boulder seems impossible. So I cleared it with my school over Christmas break and arranged to complete my thesis from 1,800 miles away, in Charlottesville. I will graduate on time.

## Early February 2001

I spend countless afternoons working on my thesis, clicking away at my laptop computer in the Charlottesville Public Library downtown, a half liter of Diet Coke snuck stealthily in my bag under the table to get me through, a warm cashmere scarf knotted around my neck to stay warm. I also have to take a couple of classes at the local community college to receive enough credit to graduate. I sit in the art history class counting calories in my notebook. I add up what I ate for breakfast, and I plan what I'll eat for lunch. And then I slowly remove every condiment, or "extra," until the meal has the lowest caloric value possible. *There,* I think to myself, *that will be an acceptable lunch: no mayonnaise, no ketchup, no dressing.* I finish tallying the calories for my day until—*Oops! I forgot to add the gum I'm chewing now.* I overestimate another handful of calories and throw that into the mix. Nothing is ever good enough.

I get a job working part-time in the nicest clothing boutique on the downtown mall, a popular, high-end store stocked with every gorgeous fabric a skinny girl like me could dream of. The walls are chock-full of beauty products and accessories; the racks hold precious pieces of fashion I never thought I would be lucky enough to own myself, even though my mother outfits herself here regularly. With my employee discount I quickly spend every extra dollar on an artful wardrobe that I have to update almost monthly because of how rapidly my body is evaporating. Eventually I realize that shopping at Old Navy is more practical: my size goes down week to week, and those several-hundred-dollar skirts and dresses I buy one month do not fit the next.

But for now I enjoy throwing my money away on clothes. I don't need money anyway. I'm staying with my mother in her small white apartment, and she pays for groceries. Most nights we eat big steamed artichokes and salads. Mom has rice, too, or chicken, but I don't. And I don't put oil on my salads like Mom does. And I don't have dessert if my little sister Tor is with us and wants some ice cream. I do have air-popped popcorn at night when we watch TV. I make a separate bowl for myself because Tor and Mom want butter on theirs.

# OCTOBER 1999

I'm a junior in college and living with Christopher. He's taken this semester off from school so that we can live together in Boulder, and he's working for a professor at CU, doing research. It's a Sunday morning, and I have slept in. When I climb out of bed, it's easy to see that the sky is full with another day of typical Boulder sunshine. Christopher is playing Ultimate Frisbee at a field on the outskirts of town, so I drive to meet him, sit on a blanket in the grass, watch him run and catch and throw. Thinking about the last twelve hours, wondering, *Is this what it means to grow up?*

When the phone rang at midnight last night, I figured quickly enough: midnight in Boulder is 2:00 A.M. back east. I first assumed it was Nat calling from Boston; he stays up late, all hours. But I heard instead my little sister Victoria's voice, crying, whispering, fearful. *I'm under the covers,* she said. *Daddy's drunk and he's screaming at Mom because she stayed out too late with Ellen.* I pictured Tor huddled in a white nightgown with her blankie, hair frayed, having been woken up in a panic, in the middle of the night. My first thought was, *I wish I was there with you right now,* my first instinct to jump on a plane. Given the age difference between us, nine and a half years, I feel like sort of a half-mother, half-sister to her. Her pain is my pain. Especially when her real mother or father can't be there for her because of whatever they are doing to each other. I feel so absent, and so scared for her.

These are the moments that we are haunted by later in life, as adults. These are the childhood moments that bring us to therapy, that we cull as "baggage" in our adult relationships. I wish Victoria wasn't having one of these moments.

*With Ellen,* my sister had said. It doesn't take a genius. I called Nat, after soothing Tor, still hearing the violent shrieks of both my parents in my head. Did they forget they had an eleven-year-old daughter in the next room? How could they forget? *She's having an affair,* I told Nat.

*My god,* he said back. *My god, you're right.*

(And so began the ripples in the landscape of our family home, the real ones, ones I could later trace into early childhood, but for now seemed to be just beginning.)

When I call my mother on Monday morning, she is subdued but graceful. *I am not,* she tells me calmly. *You know there are diseases now, Mom,* I warn. I am trying to take a reasonable approach with her, but I'm so confused. I focus on Victoria and remind my mother that she can't scream like that in front of Tor. I remind her of the pain I felt as a young girl, listening to them scream.

My parents have always fought. I remember being a little girl myself and hiding under the bed, their bed, while Mommy screamed at Daddy and Daddy slammed the door on his way out. Then the car would start and Mommy would come find me. She would pet my hair and try to soothe me, but she did it with a sad, victimized look on her face that did not help me feel any better.

*I am absolutely not having an affair,* she says again. *Then what?* I ask. *Then why?* She gives me vague, unclear answers that don't add up, and I feel crazy. Are my instincts wrong? Do parents always scream at each other in the middle of the night for no reason?

~~~

I didn't know then, I couldn't have, how much of an effect my parents' crumbling marriage would have not only in my heart, but on my body. Later I wondered if it was the simple fact that I was born of their sex, what was now broken, divided, what felt like irreparable sex—could this be what caused me to waste away? If a body is born of broken sex, how can that body thrive, even live?

Living in Colorado in 1999, I did not have an eating disorder. I did not have an exercise compulsion. I had a loyal, puppy-dog boyfriend. I had parents who took me shopping when they visited, a kid sister who loved *The Hobbit* and *The Chronicles of Narnia*. I had an older, genius brother who made me proud when he showed up in expensive clothes with beautiful women on his arm. I was a junior at Naropa University studying poetry in the lineage of Allen Ginsberg and Anne Waldman. I had interesting classes, even more interesting classmates, and a back door that opened to the foothills of the breathtaking Rocky Mountains. I had moments of anxiety, yes. But I didn't know then that anxiety is often a precursor to disorders like exercise bulimia and anorexia nervosa. I knew that when my mother was young, she had starved herself. I had known for all of my childhood that Mommy had anorexia when she was young—it was just a fact. But I did not know then that eating disorders might be genetic. I did not know then that I was capable of doing the same thing. I did not know that pain was such an unbearable thing. I did not know that my body was such a fascinating tool.

# HISTORY

My mother starved herself for a decade. She lived on cigarettes, measured coffee poured over granola, and pieces of brownie hidden under the bed in her college dorm room. She married my father when they were twenty-one, fresh out of school, just a few months after they'd met. And into the early years of marriage, my mother counted every calorie, weighed every chicken breast on her kitchen scale, split cookies in half, and said no to seconds. She didn't finish firsts.

Her recovery, as she remembers it, was gradual and unintentional. Most recovering anorexics are encouraged to gain one to two pounds each week; we joke in my family that Mom gained that little each year. But as far back as I can recollect, my mother was a reasonably normal eater. We had pancakes every Sunday morning, ice cream on summer evenings, popcorn and candy at the movies. Even though anorexia wasn't the household term in Mom's youth that it is today, she did understand, by the time she came around to raising children, that what she'd had was an eating disorder, and she didn't intend to pass it on to us.

I grew up lusty, and Mom must have breathed an internal sigh of relief, seeing me at eighteen, my round hips and belly, my boobs bouncing as I danced at concerts with friends. Charlottesville has an outdoor mall, laid in brick: the classic gathering place for families, couples, and reckless, undisciplined teenagers. I spent afternoons and evenings there, every weekend when the weather was warm, listening to the African drummers and dancing, my long hair shaking loose around my waist. During high school I had an appetite to dance, make love, sleep, and taste—rich, warm, chocolately things.

One warm spring afternoon late in my teens, we sat around the kitchen table. I remember smiling, laughing with my family, naming myself out loud a *lazy, gluttonous being.* Mom took so much pleasure in this; she still brings it up sometimes. I had realized that day, recovering from a nap, that the only things that could pull me away from sleep were either food or sex. And the only things that could pull me away from food were either sleep or sex. And that probably nothing could pull me away from sex. I didn't share this last part with my parents, but I recognized in their laughter the acceptance they felt for me, their daughter. The possibility that I could ever develop an eating disorder wasn't in question at this point: I was happy, finishing high school, dating Christopher, living and dancing and enjoying life.

I was close with Mom then, but we were closer later.

We grew closer the less I ate. We were closest driving around town, in the spring of 2001, making a deposit at the bank, picking up Tor from school, grabbing lattes around the corner from Studio 206, my mom's popular local yoga and wellness studio. We were closest then, when I was starving, when we could share clothes, when I didn't have Christopher anymore and she didn't have Dad, because they were separated. We were closest that spring, when we lived in the little white apartment on Little High Street, renting movies, eating air-popped popcorn, drinking Diet Coke, and reading *Martha Stewart Living.*

Well, I was drinking Diet Coke and reading Martha Stewart. Mom kept me company with her toast and tea, her books on meditation and new age prayer. She sat beside me on the couch that folded out into my bed and listened to me type away on my laptop as I worked to finish my college thesis from this temporary home.

When I started to gain my weight back, Mom said, *You can pass all your anorexic clothes to me!*

## FEBRUARY 21, 2001

My strict routine is morning workouts, but many afternoons I look for another chance to exercise. My mom is a sort of new age career woman, and her yoga and fitness studio downtown is beautiful. It really is. It's so *Mom:* airy, clean, lots of white space. She teaches dance classes and wears flowy pants. I go there in the evenings to take her classes, if I want a second workout. Or I just go for another run.

When people ask my mom about my dad, she tells them that she and my father are taking a break. *Fifty-two and never lived alone! Imagine that!* A sabbatical, she calls it, a respite. A little hideaway home. But some afternoons, coming home from my second run, I walk into Mom's apartment to find her crying, back pressed to the pillows at the head of her bed, knees in, whispering on the phone to her therapist. *In a minute,* she mouths to me.

I can't feel much anymore. Am I bothered by my mother's emotions? Yes. But I'm also so troubled by emotion altogether that I'm completely removed from it. In other words, I am not in touch with feeling distressed. So I continue through the apartment, climb onto the pullout sofa that doubles as my bed during the weeks that Tor stays with us and occupies the second bedroom. I am, for the most part, living with my mother. For a while I shared a house with a girl I knew from high school. But I couldn't sleep at night, and I couldn't handle being social. So after several weeks I started boarding with Mom.

Cracking open a can of Diet Coke, I turn on the TV, heading straight for the Food Network. I pull out my little recipe notebook hidden between the couch cushions and take close notes on Sara Moulton's show. Then I remake the recipe, removing all fat, sugars, and animal products, replacing any sauce or dressing with tamari or vinegar, or both, and replacing any sautéing or frying with baking and steaming. Which means that I'm left with the same meal as always: vegetables and a possible potato or grain, baked, boiled or steamed, doused in salt, vinegar, and soy sauce.

In the back of my head, I know something's wrong with Mom. When she comes out of her room she doesn't bother hiding the red from her eyes. She's dreamy and distant, and it takes hours for her to come back. When she does we go out for coffee or shopping. While Mom tells the outside world that this is a much-deserved break from living in a big house with a family and dogs and things to do, she knows I'm suspicious of a more severe cause and acknowledges at least this much to me: *An illusion has been shattered, Peach, that's all that's happened. For twenty years I held onto an illusion that I thought would save me. I know now that it won't.*

The first time she tells me this, we're driving in her BMW station wagon, heading downtown on Main Street. I get mad at her for this explanation, my skinny fingers in the air, elbows reaching outward, expressive—*Mom, what on earth, what is going on, what does that mean?*—but she has nothing else to say. And so I sink into the soft seat of Mom's car, arms falling in my lap, picturing what the shattering of an illusion might look like: white shards filling up the landscape, blinding my mother and in turn my father, keeping us all from living together, keeping me from eating.

# MARCH 2, 2001

Half the town seems to know my parents are separated, but somehow Victoria's school hasn't received the news. One particular afternoon Mom calls my cell, asking me to pick Tor up early—she's called home sick. Again. While someone goes to fetch her from class, I tromp into the administrative offices of her private middle school to say not so discreetly, *There's a reason she's been missing school. Has anyone contacted you to let you know our parents are separated? Things are not easy at home.* I have my hands on my bony hips; my head juts forward. I am so tired of protecting this: It shouldn't be a secret. But this is the genteel South, and people don't tell the truth here. People drive around in their SUVs with their coiffed hair, and they golf at the country club and smile at every party, even the party hosted by the woman who fucked your husband, or your ex who later married your best friend. People show their best, most conservative good-girl side and then slay you when you're not looking, all with a smile and freshly baked cake.

# MARCH 16, 2001

Victoria and I are together on an airplane, flying to Boston for her spring break. There is too much turbulence from Charlottesville to Dulles, as there often is on these tiny propeller planes. I'm wearing black: tight stretch jeans and a tight zip-up hoodie. My crossed legs fit comfortably in the little airplane seats. I'm in the aisle, pushing my window-seat sister to talk about our parents' separation, to not hold it in, and she's turning her head away from me, trying to read a magazine. Oddly, Mom and Dad are on their way to Bermuda, together. We are all confused, us kids, as to what they're doing there, or anywhere, together or apart. They are both working on their marriage, going to therapy together and apart, and trying to resolve their issues, whatever they are. Nat keeps his distance well enough, but Tor and I are in the middle, watching our mother pretend she hasn't been crying, watching our father eat frozen meals, going between their homes like the shuttle buses that transport us between terminals when we arrive at Dulles. The second flight, the one that takes us to Logan, is smooth, and Nat meets us in his shiny BMW, friends piled in the car.

While Nat works, Tor and I take on Boston, just us girls. She has ideas, I know, of how the day will go, and so do I: I need coffee; I need it black. I'm yelling at her, *Don't cross the street! We can't go there! Don't try that on! That's trashy! Those shoes are ugly! That's too expensive!* She wants french fries, so we tread through a sloppy Boston midday and end up sitting in a booth by the window at a family restaurant near the corner of Newbury and Exeter. I order a Diet Coke; she orders a plate of fries, bless her heart, and barely looks me in the eye.

Sitting in the restaurant, I can't even smile. I'm hungry but I don't feel it in my belly; it comes out instead in my bitchiness, ordering Tor around. She knows that something is wrong, but she doesn't talk about her feelings. She pretends she's fine; she pretends I'm fine. I pretend nothing is wrong but of course I know that I'm hungry, and that I'm grumpy, and that I'm a bad sister. I know this intellectually, but not emotionally. Not enough to soften and say to her, *I'm sorry, Victoria, that I'm such a big bitch of a big sister. I'm sorry I've been so selfish. Let's go find the fanciest restaurant on Newbury and order pie and giggle.*

We should go for cake and cocoa, get our nails done. We should pick out clothes for each other, buy matching T-shirts and bracelets, scour sales, gush over high school boys walking by. Instead, I rush her home early, back to Nat's, and I tell myself I have no idea why she is so distant.

Twelve years old, my sister. Athletic, adorable, braces and all. Adolescent, into boys, instant messaging, and teenybopper clothes. Exuberant. My sister has been a flirt since she was two years old, with her giant golden Afro of hair. She would plop onto any man's lap, touch his face, and giggle. She's brilliantly well-adjusted and adapts easily to any situation. Except, of course, how can you adapt to this one? Then there's me: twenty-one, vigilant, controlling, terrified, lonely, possessive, dominant, hateful, guilty, and cold.

The rest of vacation, I let her go. She stays up until three in the morning with Nat and his friends, drinking soda and eating ice cream, watching whatever is saved on the TiVo, chatting with friends online. I try to give her the freedom I can't give myself. I want to control her, but I can't keep her with me, I can't make her go to bed early, though I try. She is on vacation, and I am trapped inside my own head.

When we fly home, she gets juice and Chex Mix from the vending machine at the airport. I let her into the house and head straight to the gym. She must be so relieved to be home, to be away from me. When we all reunite that evening, Mom and Dad back from Bermuda, sitting on the carpet in Mom's apartment (Daddy too), they give me a Rolex watch: my mother's old watch, the one I knew had been saved for me, stashed away. My mother, my tiny mother, her watch from when she was my age, and they put it on my wrist and it slides around, too loose, and I watch their eyes and my sister. I'm sure my sister is thinking, *This family, too much is happening with this family,* and I don't know what she does all this time, all this time when the attention is on me, is on my parents, I don't know what she does because I'm not watching. I am watching instead the jewelry float around my wrist, am watching the numbers descend on the scale, am watching my face in the mirror at the gym the harder I sweat, the longer I run.

I have a regimen, and I swear by it. I wake up early every morning, as early as 5:00 A.M. if I have a morning class. Some mornings I run a six-mile loop around town. Other mornings I spend an hour on the StairMaster at the country club gym. Which is an experience to behold. The machines are packed with my parents' generation; at least half of the crowd there at any given moment has been in our house, or I have been in theirs. They know me. From time to time someone will acknowledge me, will say hello. But nobody ever utters a single concerned word about my wasting body and my ritualistic exercise behaviors. Not the trainers in the gym, or the parents of my friends. I don't blame them, really—I'm utterly unapproachable. I don't smile or make eye contact. I have not smiled in weeks, if not months. I don't reach out or welcome contact. In Boulder just a few months ago, I was steadfast at perfecting the art of being a perfect woman: I was dressing well, looking beautiful, and drinking wine. I was smiling, I had manners, ambition to marry a Harvard man and build a sweet, good-girl life. But now I'm lost in sickness and rebellion. My most frequent thought is *fuck you,* aimed at anyone standing in front of me in line, driving downtown in the lane beside me, talking about the day's news on the television, or sweating next to me on the StairMaster. My mornings are mine. My exercise is mine. *If you talk to me, you motherfucking asshole bitch-faced southern snob, I swear to god I will kick you in the face and enjoy it.* Not the healthiest thought, but I'm consumed these days with anger and fear.

Despite Bermuda and whatever it meant, Daddy goes back home to the big house and Mom stays in her pristine white apartment. I stay with her. Spring slowly lurches forward, our family twisting, unable to bud, though watching leaves all around us slowly sprout. By April we have warm weather and Samuel, my therapist, asks me one afternoon if I am enjoying any part of early spring.

I have been in therapy with Samuel since I came home in January. We talk a little bit about my body and how I feel about it. How I feel about food. But mostly we talk about my parents, or about Christopher. I love Samuel. I love his office, his face, his beard, his deep, gentle voice. I love his leather sofa and his unbelievably casual way of working. He puts his feet up and eats pretzels or sucks on lollipops. He is like a grandfather to me. I feel safer here than anywhere.

*Spring?* I think. *I haven't really noticed.* I am wearing a big wool sweater. It must be seventy degrees outside, but my body temperature is always below zero. *Is it spring?*

# APRIL 2001

My dreams lately are following a theme. I wake up every morning with visions of the previous night's drama: sex, death, sometimes the two combined, always with childhood friends or ex-boyfriends, often with Christopher. But I'm not so disturbed by them. My life feels fateful—a sad fate, but everything is in proper order. So I'm dreaming death and murder. *Makes sense,* I think to myself. That's about how things feel these days: My life is falling apart and I'm clutching the edges to hold myself up. The dreams, I believe, are my insides forcing themselves out.

April 3, 2001

The Dogwood Festival will be later this month, and I picture being happy, even laughing. Or maybe by my 22nd birthday in Greece I'll have laughed. And maybe one day Christopher will decide to love me again. Or maybe I'll become a kid again. Or move to the tropics, Hawaii, Bali? Or maybe I'll never marry. Maybe I'll write a novel. Start a women's poetry group. Make a million on the granola recipe. Move to Paris and be dark and thin. Stay always in Virginia with a pickup truck and snap peas growing in the garden. Teach yoga at Studio 206. Move to Louisiana for my husband's job. Start a restaurant. Decorate homes. Run a marathon. Dream my life away. Write a thousand memories. Make art books. Return home. Call out.


April 4, 2001

Dreamt last night that I went to Mom's friend for help on my thesis but instead she gave me life advice, telling me that pleasure will come only from what is innate to day-to-day living—first morning breaths, peeing, etc. In other words, simplify.

It could be a good day.

April 8, 2001

I can't get last night's dream out of my head. In a bed—this bed, my bed—with Christopher. We're asleep. In the night I roll his body on top of mine, wanting him to be with me again through using my body. Now he's naked. Very heavy on top of me. My arm on his broad, Christopher shoulder. I think he's bigger than in real life. A little. We're having sex but in sleep state. It's too much for me. I try to push him off but he's too heavy. Image of my palm pushing his pelvis away and it twisting slightly but he stays inside me. Ejaculates. No condom. I'm upset, I have a pinky liquid pooling from me. Blood mixed with semen. But I'm not in physical pain. I go to the bathroom, come back and am still pooling this mixture. Christopher looks handsome but unusually intense—eyes at their bluest and his teeth tinted this same color. I start to freak out, tell him I'm not on the pill anymore, and how could he have done this—I'd been trying to push him off. I panic and bombard him with questions: Did he practice safe sex with the last girl he slept with? He tells me yes and not to worry, but something here isn't right. He's not being gentle or sweet. Not quite irritated either, just uncaring. He leaves as the phone rings.

My relationship with my mother is deepening, becoming the primary relationship in my life right now. I am learning so much, like how strikingly different (and similar) the dynamics are from a relationship of lovers. Mom and I do get jealous and dependent, but we're more willing and much more understanding about separating from each other. Much less possessive. Much less fearful. I don't really worry about losing her love, so there is a freedom in that. There is the sense that I love my mother purely and self-lessly enough that I really want her to be happy, to have what she craves. Even when I can't be a part of it.


April 9, 2001
OK, I'll admit it. It's getting "worse," and it's a surpris-ingly rapid fall. I've had so much energy these days. Food doesn't seem to give me energy—it is coming from elsewhere. I don't need to eat. I feel great! But I know I'm getting pretty thin, and no, I don't know if I know how to stop—how to level my weight instead of continuing to lower my calorie count. It's a totally addictive and obsessed thing. "Just a little more." An interesting thing: I get very few hunger pangs.


April 12, 2001
Mom talks about when she had anorexia—that she was dying and she chose life. Is it really possible to die this way? So painless. Now everybody tells me I look thin. It's mostly in my arms and chest. Sometimes I see the disease in myself. Sometimes I still see fat in my thighs. I

have no butt or hips anymore, just bony buttons, pro-
truding knobs.


April 17, 2001
Dreamt last night of being in a scary movie with Jack
Nicholson, where Christopher was laughing maniacally
across the aisle of a train when I told him I loved him
still.
       I can't even imagine kissing. Not Christopher or
anyone. Can't even see it.


April 18, 2001
Dreamt last night of a grade-school classmate forcing sex
on me, and trying to do the same to one of my friends,
who was somewhat asleep.


April 19, 2001
I think another violent or unpleasant sex dream last
night, but I don't remember details. Oh yes—a gun ex-
ploding in the front seat of my pickup truck while I was
inside with my lover, not sure who he was. Also a scene at
a ski slope. The guy at the chairlift asked me to drop and
give him ten. Smugly and easily, I did more pushups than
he asked for as if to prove him wrong—prove me strong.

April 23, 2001
Dreamt last night that Christopher died.


April 27, 2001
I want to be thinner. At the dentist the receptionist told me, You're tiny! I wasn't that small when I was born! But I think people I know are getting used to my little size and have stopped remarking. All the "You look scary" comments have stopped. I haven't gained a pound. At the gym this morning I weighed myself. Smallest I've ever been. I think people are adjusting. I've been doing about 1,200 calories/day. Think I'll try out 1,100.


April 30, 2001
In my dream last night three men were after me. The first was my old lover Derek. He kept trying to have sex with me, and I didn't want to. I kept saying, Can't you just hold me? The second tried to win me over by letting me use his sculpture to turn in for my final art project. I kept saying, I need to do it for myself. I don't remember much about the third.

# APRIL 25, 2001

It's predawn. I'm sitting on a pillow, listening to bird beaks break into the sky; somehow they know light is coming and I must, too, because I've been waking up at this hour for several days in a row. My body, despite the lack of nourishment, has boundless energy. My limbs, now model-long (somehow they seem longer now that they are thinner), hang from the chair as I sip morning tea in my dance clothes, waiting for the light to advance so that I can go downtown with Mom, to her studio, to dance and weave with other women, women who now look enormous to me in their roomy thighs and generous masses of stomach.

I don't hide my weight. It's still spring, but we've had a week of summer hot weather. I sat downtown yesterday in tiny spandex shorts and a bra top, scribbling in my journal, knowing somehow that I would be offensive—that or sexy. The two are confused in my mind, not knowing which is my intention, which I want.

# MAY 2, 2001

I think I know my aim. I've told my family I'm making a feminist statement: That's what this weight loss is about, Mom. It's a study. I'm doing a study; I'm using my body as an example. I only look like a whore to show you what you get when you tell a girl she must be *this* or *that* or anything, really. You want thin, do you? You want sexy? You want an available woman? You want her to please you? Well, open your eyes, men of my land, feast them on my body. No? Don't want to look? You didn't mean *that* skinny? You meant for me to do it differently? This is for you, you hot, sweaty Virginia man, catcalling in the night, in the afternoon, as I walked down the street when I was twelve, or fifteen, or seventeen. This is for you, Father, Mother, who had ideas for my adulthood before I was born. This is for you, every woman's clothing store that doesn't extend beyond a size 10. This is for you, friend from high school who ran twice a day to burn your body down and skipped dessert. This is for you, my brother, who is successful in other ways, ways I can't be, ways that so far remove yourself from our family. This is for you, Christopher. You thought I couldn't take on a challenge. You thought I couldn't do it on my own.

My parents don't know what to make of me. They are concerned, and they show it differently. Mom has started talking about *treatment*. Daddy and I don't see much of each other; I think he avoids me, and that's his way of letting me know something is really wrong. Mom doesn't buy my "feminist statement" argument, but she listens.

I'm wearing lace camisoles as shirts and miniskirts (in fluorescent orange or denim) rising so high that if I had any flesh left on my backside, it would peek out below. I'm wearing high heels and have long, red, fake nails glued to my own, done by the nail technician at the mall one recent afternoon as I clutched a half liter of Diet Coke. I shelled out a small tip, adjusting to this strange new length in my fingers. In my whole body, really. I'm a novelty even to myself.

# MAY 8, 2001

I call Mom one evening to say *Meet me at Old Navy!* She does, and we're in the dressing room together trying on jeans. I laugh a lot when I'm shopping: I love shopping! I love buying clothes! I love that I'm a size 0 everywhere and fit into the kids clothes in some stores. Mom suddenly looks upset and says to me, *I'll meet you at home; I have to go.* It ruins my shopping binge, and I leave without buying anything. When I get home, she's sitting alone at the kitchen table.

*What, Mom?* She tells me to sit beside her. She has this terrible, crumbling look on her face, like she's disappointed herself or me or something. *We've hired a team of doctors,* she tells me. And in a way, it's everything I've dreamed of, but suddenly I'm scared. I've been screaming for attention, but I don't really want it. Or I do. Or I don't know. Do I have an eating disorder? Am I going to get help? Mom says she's talked with Samuel, and he agrees that I need more help. She has hired *specialists,* she tells me. A dietitian. A second therapist. And an actual physician. I have to go to the actual doctor starting next week. They are going to weigh me and make me pee into a cup. Twice a week. Really?

But first we have to throw a party. My diploma is on its way, in the mail, and I planned my own graduation party months ago.

# MAY 12, 2001

My eating disorder is in her heyday—this is the height of my control. I have my intake down to a bare minimum, and I'm running religiously, beyond religiously, devoutly. I have a system down pat: snacking on pickles, celery, and salsa and fixing huge dinners that fill the plate with lettuce and chopped-up veggie burgers, all spritzed with vinegar and soy sauce. I have even discovered how to incorporate some treats while keeping within my calorie limitations. I found the best fat-free brownies at a local health food store, and I top them with just enough peanut butter to taste it. If I eat one-quarter of this dessert concoction, it costs me only a small number of calories: less than half an apple.

I'm flaunting my skinny body while I preach my feminist study, and I'm relishing the dazzling glory of my tiny, tiny frame. I love high heels. I love dresses. I'm dancing in my accomplishment, proud of the lines in my bony face, boastfully showcasing my long, straight thighs.

(I will recognize later that life is a series of fleeting moments: Everything is temporary, and this phase certainly was. I could not maintain the behaviors that were ensuring this thin form. I could not maintain such excessive exercise. I could not maintain such a low caloric intake.)

I delight in my achievement. I think I am the envy of every one of my friends. And so I throw a party at my parents' big house. I have it catered. I call the party in my name. And I buy a new dress.

I order my dress from a catalog. Blue feels right for a summer party, airy and upbeat, and I need all the boost I can get. I don't know it, though, thinking I look my best ever this evening as I'm getting ready. Mom sent me to the salon for an updo this morning, and I came back with my head looking even more disproportionately huge next to my body, now that my waist-length hair is piled on top.

This is my graduation party. I designed the invitations myself, complete with the Naropa University seal, and sent them to everyone I could think of: friends who were back in town from college, families I'd known most of my life, and my brother, who flew down from Boston with his two best friends, Matt and Mark. I passed them eating Mexican food downtown this morning while I was on my way to get my hair done. They looked happy and easeful, until they spotted me and waved nervously as I walked by, probably grateful that I didn't stop to talk.

I went with Mom this morning to pick them up from the airport. Nat did his best to fake a smile as we hugged, and I did my best to look chipper. I am, in fact, thrilled to see him, though I know my body is different now, and I know it is hard for other people to pretend. But I want them to see what I see—a happy, pretty, determined young woman.

(It is during this month, with all these homecomings, seeing old friends, that my distorted perspective will begin to shift. What I have deemed lovely, lean, and strong, I begin to recognize that others see as sick, weak, and even insane.)

I was wearing a ruby ring when we went to fetch Nat at the airport, given to me this morning by my mother, a gift from her and my aunt. It looked so tiny in the box but fit my hand perfectly, delicate, gold like my hair, and deep red—like blood, I thought, though I have none of that, not recently, not for some time.

Nat didn't know how to react. He tried to behave normally, I could tell, but in that way that someone acts when they're clearly *trying* to act normally but feel incredibly awkward. He avoided a real hug, and instead we drifted into a sort of leaned-in shoulder pat. He had his friends Matt and Mark to buffer him, and they behaved similarly: hesitant.

Now that I'm up in my attic bathroom applying mascara and perfume, ready to walk down the stairs grandly like a princess to greet my guests, I feel all the anticipation I imagine I'll feel on my wedding day. The attention is going to be on me, and I am stunning, in the true sense of the word. And blind to my own disease, blind to how I really look, blind to what I've done, though I've felt so in control since the beginning.

Casey is the first to arrive. We're best friends from middle school, but she's a year behind me, in school in Southern California. She's sunburned from a day of hiking with her father, looking plump to me in something trendy, her hair cut short. She comes up to my room and I want her to admire me, to be jealous of how beautiful I am, to fawn and coo over my dress and hair. She doesn't, though; instead, she gives me the same fake smile Nat gave me in the airport, the same fake smile she gave me last week, the night we reunited, after which, staring me dead in the eyes, she'd said, *You look gaunt, Peach, sick. I had no idea it had gone this far.*

I spend the next few hours greeting guests with smiles and hugs as they bring boxes with bows and bottles of champagne, watching all these friends fill our big hollow house with their cheeks red from drinking and late spring nights, caterers drifting through from the kitchen, Dad's party rule being fastidiously followed: Never let a guest's wine glass remain empty. I stand for one stolen moment on the side porch, looking over the long stairs that glide down the hill of my parents' side yard and by the brick fountain where my mother is standing. I'm watching her, her hair and hands in the air, my mother, my mother, wishing I could still the moment, take her with me, my mother and her hair—before someone comes up behind me and I'm wrapped back into conversation, woven into the night, through all the rooms of our big house, into the air, bubbles and smoke everywhere but in my own mouth. I will drink nothing but air.

It's the end of the night, and most guests have left, except for those who always stay late at Friedman parties: our best friends, the couples I've seen drunk in my parents' living room since I was a girl; and my friends, my generation, easing back into cushy chairs and fingering stems of final champagne glasses, maybe a lingering cigarette. I begin to open my gifts. Delicate pieces of jewelry emerge: pearls laid in gold on a gemstone chain; hanging, precious earrings; gentle pink beads strung on thin elastic. I'm slipping everything onto my body, drunk on the attention, on the people sitting in my living room, late on an early summer night, watching me finally retreat into the kitchen to eat two chicken breasts and a lemon square.

I cannot believe I've done it. The party has gone so late that it's disrupted my eating routine. I haven't been able to eat my typical dinner or to go to bed early to stave off any more hunger. All night caring, gentle voices have whispered in my ear, *Darling, I am worried about you,* and so, for the first time after months of calculated portions and predetermined meal planning, I eat food. Catered food. Food cooked for taste, not control. And it tastes. Unbearably good. So good that when all the guests leave, when I am finally alone on the first floor of the house, I grab a bag of jelly beans, and I eat them. And a leftover brownie from the dessert tray. And another lemon bar.

And then. In fear that I will never stop, I pull my bony arm from reaching any farther and carry myself up two flights of stairs and into my attic bedroom.

On the way I think back four days, to the moment when my mother sat me down at the kitchen table and told me she was staging a medical intervention. Starting next week, I'll have daily doctors' appointments, sometimes twice daily. When she told me, I was frozen. And then I blushed, I giggled, but I didn't cry. I'm thinking about this now, as I'm dragging myself away from the lemon squares and chicken breasts. I'm thinking, *I'm not ready to make a change;* I'm thinking, *This isn't symbolic, this isn't a crossroads, this isn't a turning point, no, please.*

I fall asleep dazzlingly hungry, my lips wet with want. Tomorrow, I promise myself, dozing off with my updo still in place, a million bobby pins poking at my scalp, I will be back on track: lettuce with vinegar, one veggie patty, and popcorn before bed. Maybe an apple.

# MAY 15, 2001

It's the time of year when friends are reuniting—returning home from school or semesters abroad—and I haven't been sure about how to anticipate my own reunions. I've been able to keep my eating disorder somewhat hidden from my out-of-town friends, and as a rule I'm fairly antisocial these days. But after my graduation party, when so many people came to see me, and when I finally let myself be seen, suddenly my body is the buzzword on the street. Some friends are responding politely. Some are responding with fear. But my friend Lily—she's got nothing to give but love.

The thing about Lily: She's kind of amazing. I mean that. I can tell her anything. She is the most nonjudgmental, generous, kind friend I have ever had. She is not afraid of me or my eating disorder. She is not angry with me for losing weight or getting sick. She is scared, but she doesn't show it to me. Instead, she offers to help, and I let her.

So it's Lily who takes me by the hand, her beautiful head of shiny, curly hair, and drives me to my first appointment with Anne, my new dietitian. For several months Lily and I have been planning a summer trip to Europe: France, Italy, and Greece, as a celebration of our college graduation. But it's become clear that I won't be able to go. I went to the travel agency this past week and cancelled my ticket, then told Lily that I won't be going with her. She wasn't surprised. I can sort of recognize that I'm missing out on an awesome opportunity because something is wrong with me. So wrong that staying home, depressed, with my mother and working on losing weight sounds more appealing than going to Europe. In fact, it's the only thing that seems manageable to me. That, and sitting by the pool with a trashy romance novel. I've told everyone that's how I'm spending my summer. I can't wait, but I'm a little disappointed that I don't get to smoke cigarettes and wear my black dresses in Greece.

I'm nervous on our way to Anne's. Lily takes me for lunch at Subway first—a rarity for me, but I know I can get safe food there—and I order vegetables with vinegar on bread. And Diet Coke! Thank god for Diet Coke. When we finally arrive at Anne's, she opens the door, looks directly at me standing behind Lily, and ushers me into her office. I think to myself, *How does she know that I'm the patient, and not Lily?* I can't see how different our bodies look. I mean, Lily and I are both thin. Maybe I'm a little thinner, but is it that noticeable?

Anne's office is in her home. She leads me through the living room, where Lily sits down with a book to read, and into her office. I settle into a comfortable leather chair opposite Anne and try to take everything in. I look around the room at her diplomas and her posters about food, exercise, and wellness. I look up at Anne and notice how pretty she is, how young she looks, how healthy and happy and energetic she seems. And then, as she starts to ask questions, I look down at my hands until, before I know it, I'm opening up.

I talk to Anne about my fears of food. I start to cry. It's the first emotion I've let come out in months. I tell her about the chicken and the lemon squares. I tell her that I don't need to learn to eat, that I need to learn to not eat, because if I'm given permission to eat, I won't stop. *I know they're worried I have anorexia, but actually I eat too much,* I tell her.

Anne cuts into me like I soon cut into cakes: determined, impassioned, and frequent. She explains what I've done to myself physiologically, metabolically. She is worried about my food intake and extremely worried about my exercise. She encourages me to stop working out immediately and cautions that I could have a heart attack at any moment. She explains the notion of metabolic shutdown—this is when the body begins to conserve calories, when the body's metabolism slows dramatically, as a response to being under-fueled and overworked. She tells me that I will die if I don't change my behavior. I'm still observing Anne and trying to figure her out. She is really pretty. She is young, probably only a few years older than me. She is tan, blonde, athletic. Immediately I like her. No, I want to be like her. I want to do well by her, to recover for her. As I leave she gives me homework for this first week: I have to eat three snacks a day and cut my workouts in half. Minimum.

Lily walks me out of Anne's office with a meal plan in hand. We cross the street to Lily's car, and I'm utterly confused, scared, excited, or just unsure how to feel at all. Meeting Anne was a little bit like being back in junior high and seeing the cool girl you want to be friends with. I want her to like me. I feel inspired. I feel changed. Sort of. Maybe. For a second, a half a second, maybe. But maybe not changed enough to add three snacks a day and cut my workouts in half. I want to be healthy again. Will being healthy mean being like Anne? I can stomach the idea of being like Anne. I can maybe, possibly, momentarily imagine being like her. If that is healthy, maybe, maybe I'll try.

~~~

There are so many countless moments, hundreds of them, thousands, about which I can say, *This is when I decided to get better* or *This is when I knew I was going to make a change.* There are thousands of these moments because it's a process, a long process involving hundreds and thousands of steps. But some moments stand out, and meeting Anne was one of them.

# MAY 18, 2001

Catherine is the best-known eating disorder therapist in town. I met with her once before, when I was fifteen and undergoing my first round of therapy because my grades were bad. I didn't like her then; something about the way she looked at me and talked to me made me self-conscious, so I chose a younger, long-haired therapist with an exotic name: Sandra Carillo. I didn't have an eating disorder then; I don't really know why we tried Catherine, but maybe there were signs of the problems to come even before I knew it.

It's six years later now, nearly seven. I'm twenty-one and back in Catherine's office, one week after my graduation party. Samuel, the therapist I love who has watched me waste away, thinks I need to see a specialist, too. And Anne agrees. Catherine is a specialist. Catherine has groups, they tell me. Groups. I can be in a group.

Mom comes with me. We sit side by side and Catherine tells me the road to recovery is long. I like her now; she's sympathetic and gentle. I like that she's older than me, older than my mother. I study her body, but bodies confuse me lately. I can't tell if she's fat or thin. I can't tell but I like her eyes. I like sitting in her office; it's a different office from when I was fifteen, but it's in the same neighborhood. Everything in Charlottesville is in this neighborhood: the ear-nose-throat specialist I saw as a child, the dermatologist I saw as an adolescent, and the vacuum repair shop with the man who took me out for a margarita when I was eighteen.

Catherine says that a secure home life could help me recover. Then they ask me to leave the room; Mom wants to tell Catherine something in private. She has that funny look—how can I put my finger on it? It says, *Darling girl, there are still things you can't know. Darling girl, I have to tell the doctor something you can't know. Darling.* So I go into the waiting room and look at pamphlets. I'm wearing a miniskirt and I think my legs are so beautiful. I'm happy to be here. When they call me back in, there is some condescending smiling that feels really nice. It feels comforting to be treated like a child. Catherine asks me if it's okay that I had to leave the room for a bit and I say, *Oh yes, there are some things I can't know.*

# MAY 26, 2001

It's been just over a week that we've all been back in the big house together, Mom abandoning her little white apartment to come home, I think because my doctors said it would be best to look like a happy family. I have almost two weeks of treatment under my belt, and Mom went in to meet with my therapists without me there. I'm not gaining any weight; in fact, I'm still losing, but I've tried, I swear I have, to make changes. I just. Can't.

I have moved myself comfortably onto the third floor of the big house, decorated a small living room of my own, and packed a tidy mini-kitchen in a corner of my bedroom. I spend nights reading thick, romantic novels and eating air-popped popcorn.

I've been trying to get a tan, but I can't figure out why my body won't take the sun. I lie out topless in the backyard (even when Dad pulls his car down the driveway) with a Diet Coke on ice, swishing the gnats away. The grass is itchy; I can't get comfortable. I shift the little bottom half of my swimsuit from side to side, wondering how long I have to lay out to get any color. I can't figure out why I'm so pale, or why my fingernails are purple. I've noticed white hair growing soft and delicate all over my face and body, but I haven't been able to link that to my skimpy diet. (As it turns out, this hair, called lanugo, grows when the body is underweight as a means of insulation since so much fat has been lost.)

People turn away from me now. Walking into the supermarket earlier today, I tried making eyes at an attractive, slightly older man. He looked away so quickly. And friends don't let their gazes linger either; that is, the few friends I'm forced to see when I venture out in public with my mother. Last night we went to Barnes and Noble for coffee and browsing, and I saw a girl from high school. She looked me straight in the eyes, hugged me, asked about our mutual pregnant friend. I told Mom, as we walked out, *She didn't even notice . . .* I'm aware that friends don't want to look at my body, but then I'm disappointed when they don't show any concern. Mom said, *Honey, nobody knows what to say.* I wonder about that now, lying out in the yard in my new black bikini. (By the next summer, I will have handed my tiny bathing suits down to my budding, beautiful sister, who wears them with the perfect amount of luscious early teenage flesh.)

~~~

When I look back at these moments of my illness—particularly the sense that I was so aware of what I was doing, that I knew I was starving myself, that it was a feminist study—I'm flooded with sensation. I look at my body now, in what feels like different skin and flesh, and watch my hairs stand on end. *It's scary.* It's scary what I did to myself. And it's scary how I justified it—a feminist study!? Who were you kidding, Peach? On the one hand, I understand what I meant then. I did have some degree of consciousness about my eating disorder. I did know that I was angry at men, at the media, and with my family. I knew that starving and overexercising provided an escape, a way to distance myself from my emotions. But I did not know, or see, or understand, how much I was hurting myself. I did not understand how much work recovering from these habits would require. I did not understand that being angry and acting out was actually easier than learning to treat myself well, to care for myself, to nourish myself through the heartache I felt so deeply. That understanding took time.

## MAY 28, 2001

The big wooden back door of my parents' house is open, the screen just slammed shut, and I'm in the kitchen with the white phone cord wrapped around my arms. Mom and Dad are eating on the patio to give me privacy with the intake nurse from a hospital in Georgia. It's dinnertime. I'm supposed to eat potatoes with Parmesan cheese.

I've eaten even less than usual since my graduation party two weeks ago. Despite my new doctor's input, despite my moments of desire to be well, despite Anne's inspiration, I've battled my body back into submission, lost another couple of pounds so that I'm my lowest ever, at around one hundred pounds. I've also put in a few extra minutes at the gym every day on the StairMaster, surviving on diet ice-pops, buying them by the case from Kmart, keeping them in the mini-freezer right by my bed. Luckily my sister and my friend Lily like them, too: We spend a couple hours shoveling them down our throats and giggling the afternoon after my party, when Lily brings over a video from my twenty-first birthday, which she spent with me in Colorado eleven months before. I notice how happy I look on her tape: drunk, sexy, middle of the night full of life midsummer in Boulder, just one year before. Here I am now, turning twenty-two in less than a month, shriveled away, trapped in my attic bedroom with socks on my toes to keep warm.

The intake nurse says to me, on the phone, *Well, that sounds very healthy,* after I tell her I had a turkey sandwich for lunch. I don't tell her it was on forty-calorie bread with one slice of turkey, one slice of lettuce, one slice of tomato. I don't tell her I've lost weight since I started outpatient treatment, that I've been interpreting my dietitian's meal plan in my own way. I don't tell her the granola bar she's applauding as a snack was the smallest, lowest-fueling kind I could find in the store. Instead, I nod on the other end of the phone, say *Thank you,* with my knees hugging my chest, feet and sit bones pressing against the wicker of my mother's desk chair, back pressing into the slabs behind.

I am not trying to deceive her. I am not trying to manipulate. I am being honest in my own confusion and self-deprecation. I *did* eat a turkey sandwich, and to stop and tell her my whole lunch was less than a hundred calories feels like unnecessary boasting. *These doctors at the hospital in Georgia work with anorexics all day long,* I tell myself. *She must know I don't mean one of those turkey sandwiches from the deli.* But her praise for my food choices inspires guilt: *I have not been a good enough anorexic. I have eaten too much; my meals sound normal.* She notes that my weight is low; she expresses concern when I tell her about my body hair, the white furry patches growing on my face and shoulders. I am honest that I haven't had my period in several months, that the scab on my finger hasn't healed from March, that the skin under my nails is always purple. We hang up and I think, *I can't go to the hospital, they won't let me exercise there, I bet they won't let me exercise there.*

It's a blur, what I do now, whether I am wearing the blinding orange hooded sweatshirt and denim miniskirt or a pair of my little sister's shorts and a tube top. It's a blur, whether my hair is up or down, whether I've put on lipstick today. Is it a weekend or the middle of the week? Am I wearing shoes? Flip-flops? It's a blur because I know I'm about to do something drastic. My adrenaline starts to pump, the blood rushes to my head, and I feel a level of rising pressure and excitement that's so strong I lose some of my ability to focus on details or pay attention to my surroundings. But suddenly I'm taking my mother aside, we're whispering, it's important nobody knows, and then we're in the car and before I can think about it any harder I'm eating a waffle cone from Ben and Jerry's, the terror shrill on my skin and in my ears it's deafening what I'm doing but there we have it, cream on my lips chocolate down my throat my mother too sitting in the car we had to hide my limbs so long we'd make a spectacle now finished in just a few minutes more calories inside my belly than a typical day's diet what, what am I doing, what have I done.

Later that evening, I sit on the step outside the back door, watching the rain. I'm trying desperately to calm myself, because suddenly my body feels out of control. Since the ice cream just a couple of hours before, my metabolism has gone on overdrive—hunger sirens are wailing. I remember feeling this way after my graduation party, after I ate the chicken breasts and lemon squares. This is the key to being an anorexic: *You cannot eat!* Once you do, it's impossible to stop, the body responds so quickly, demanding more. Folded forward, holding my feet in my hands, I want to keep eating; I'm salivating and my belly is growling. Fighting my hunger, the strangeness of feeling so tempted, so out of control, I take a drive in my truck, buy a pack of cigarettes, the lightest I can find, and a Diet Coke. When the rain starts I maneuver my way back to Mom and Dad's house, sit there on the step as the water falls like a sheet just in front of me, off the roof and down the patio, into the grass. I know my mother comes out to soothe me. I know the panic in my face is fierce. I know I wait for them to go to bed before I begin to eat what will become the most memorable binge of my recovery: the way cashews taste when you are starved, the weight of honey on my tongue, salty crackers with peanut butter and chocolate-covered cookies. Next, spoonfuls of mint-chip ice cream, stale pretzels, leftover pasta, lemonade, sesame candies, and, finally, more cashews. Then a pear.

Mom has to help me up the stairs; I'm beside myself. She stays in bed with me until I fall asleep, which takes a while considering the extraordinary stretch I've given my belly, the rumbling and the pain. She is worried I will purge, or worse try to hurt myself some other way, but I don't—I don't even want to, the discomfort so excruciating I only want to lie in my bed and let it pass. Or maybe perch by the window with a cigarette, blowing smoke out the window, pitching the butt onto the roof, watching it get caught between the squares of slate or maybe fall into the copper gutters designed to catch rain.

Tonight, though, I can't smoke. I can't do anything but moan into Mommy's armpit, make her swear to me that I'll be okay, and she does, petting my sweaty face, holding me close to her chest and I think, *I once fit inside her, this woman, this little woman. I fit inside her belly; I lived there.* She shushes me, rubs my body, I can tell is thrilled inside that I have eaten something, that perhaps the spell is breaking, but simultaneously frightened by my extremes, how I let myself binge so heavily after such routine restriction. She is worried for my whimpering mouth, furrowed forehead, worried for how I will recover. She has had quiet conversations with my doctors; I have heard her weave into the other room with the phone cord, close the door behind her; I have seen her smile falsely to my face when she comes back in, return the phone to its carriage, go on to some daily task. She is taking time off work, my mother, for me. For me, though my sister is twelve and a half, though my sister has just spent six months floating between my mother and father's separate houses, though my sister will get her first period in less than a year, though my sister is adolescent and needs a mother it is I who am demanding parental attention. Who even knows where my sister is, what she is doing, while I am bony and holding in mountains of food, my mother petting me to sleep.

~~~

There were many memorable binges in my refeeding, but this one, no pun intended, took the cake. I tried, every day for a while, to starve myself again, but I no longer could. I was pulled toward food like a lover to her mate, sirens wailing, desperate, growling. I needed to eat. What I embarked on was a confused relationship with food. I loved it. I wanted it. It made me feel horny, sexy, wet. It did, it really did. I tell friends that and they're dumbfounded or disgusted, but really, I sat on the floor some afternoons spooning peanut butter from jars, and wow—it was juicy like sex, I swear. But I also cursed my food. My addiction, my dependence on exercise, heightened as I loosened my grip on my appetite and let food, lots of rich, decadent food, slip past my lips and into my mouth. My doctors allowed me to stay in Charlottesville; I didn't have to be hospitalized—I was gaining weight. I know the fear of the hospital in Georgia, where I wouldn't be able to exercise, is part of what got me to eat and keep eating. In Georgia, in a hospital, I would have to both eat and relinquish control of working out. *If I stay home,* I told myself, *I know I can trick my doctors. I can gain weight. I'll trick everyone, I'll trick my family, too. I'll eat; I'll gain weight. But I won't stop working out.*

I was, in fact, getting pats on the back from everyone now but Anne—Anne, who realized that my exercise bulimia was worsening as my anorexia was improving. I was gaining weight, I was eating, but I was married even more than before, if that was possible, to my exercise regimen. I had added in squats and a walk before dinner. Instead of smoking and napping in the afternoons, I was pitching in at home to help Mom reorganize the house, so that I could run up and down sets of stairs and carry boxes. I was doing cartwheels in the yard to burn calories and standing up as much as possible. My fear of weight gain was deep, and while it was bound to happen considering the amount of food I was eating, the thought of adding pounds to my skeleton still terrified me. Every run became a little longer, until finally I reached nearly ten miles. Plus those afternoon squats.

# JUNE 8, 2001

He picks me up at my house. He knocks on that big, fat door like he had so many times in high school. Other times in high school he threw rocks: My window was visible from the street; I kept my light on. He threw rocks or pennies and I went downstairs and my hair was long and we kissed or held hands or sat in the kitchen on the marble countertops and he ate from the fridge.

This time he knocks. I'm not supposed to love him anymore, or anyone, I'm anorexic, I'm a compulsive exerciser, I just started treatment recently, I've just started bingeing every night, and when he shows up he has a box of doughnuts in the car and I eat maybe four or five. And then I want a cigarette, I want a cigarette now and a Diet Coke now, and he has one in the car—a cigarette—which is strange because nobody smokes but he says it was a friend's or I don't question it, and I light the cigarette and his brother is in the back and says *Since when do we let people smoke in the car* and I could care less and Christopher seems like he could care less, too, and so I smoke it and it feels good with the window down, the late spring or early summer, that time between seasons in Virginia when it's hot enough to be called summer but the calendar says it's not quite, I guess, so we drive to the minigolf course like we did in high school, like what, are we trying to reenact something? Are we trying to fall in love again?

When he knocked on the door a few minutes ago and I went outside we walked down the walk to his car he reached for my hand, that's all I remember, I don't remember if I took it or not I can't imagine that I did he isn't mine I'm not really much of a body anyway I don't have much of a hand but he reached for it and I imagine I didn't let him really hold my hand though now I wonder what he wanted with that reach, the old Peach back, the one whose hand was soft and not nearly so skinny?

At the minigolf course we try to play but I'm inept. I can't be with people all I talk about is food and my body I can really only see inside myself though I'm sure the minigolf course is orange like it always has been and I'm sure he is nervous and his brother doesn't much know what to say and I don't know where the night goes. I don't remember being dropped off back at home and I don't remember hugging.

But I do remember high school, and playing minigolf with our friends, and how happy my parents were that I hung out with kids who played minigolf instead of the kids I used to hang out with. In high school we'd lie across the course and turn cartwheels, and Christopher and I were probably too nervous to kiss but we loved each other from across the course in a very nervous way, and once or twice I got a hole in one, but primarily I laughed and made noise and ran around feeling pretty lucky and alive.

It isn't like that anymore even if you're with the same boy who looks slightly more like a man and the same brother who also looks slightly older but you look twenty years older and your body really is gone along with your personality and you don't care about swinging a putter or the people you used to love at this point you probably just want to get home and go to bed I wonder how I felt about those doughnuts I think I felt pretty full.

# JUNE 14, 2001

Finally my twenty-second birthday arrives. Mom and I go to the Outer Banks of North Carolina, alone, for five nights. It's a peaceful trip, as I'm removed from almost all stressors and life is pared down to just me, Mom, and the ocean. I eat ice cream cones on the boardwalk and shrimp cocktail on restaurant patios. We go for beauty treatments at the spa in the afternoon and running in the morning. At least, I run in the morning. We share a room, and I sleep okay.

We take a lot of photographs; I'm obsessed with photographs. A couple weeks ago I made my friend Jane take black and whites of me naked, by the waterfall on her parents' property. I could feel my willpower beginning to diminish then, at the start of treatment. I needed a record of how my body looked— my body, which I was beginning to see as fantastic, awesome, and amazing, in the real sense of those words.

I still want a record of it, because now at the beach I've gained a few pounds, and I look quite skinny but less deathly. Mom and I buy matching pajamas at a little beach boutique: They are beautiful, expensive, extremely soft, thin cotton pajamas with yellow ribbon laced through for detail around the edges. We take photographs of ourselves in matching pajamas in our hotel room.

On my birthday night I don't want cake. Mom is nervous about how to broach that subject. I don't want fancy food either. Just shrimp cocktail by the beach, no real celebration or recognition. I am twenty-two, I am with my mother, I am slowly beginning to heal. Slowly.

# JUNE 24, 2001

Back from the beach, in Charlottesville, I can't find that sense of peace that I had, in moments, alone with Mommy on the Outer Banks. I feel spastic, panicked, tangled.

I've already run once today. This morning. Anne wants me to slow it to a walk; she wants me to cut the time at least in half. Anne actually wants me to stop exercising altogether but I can't. This is the reason I didn't go to the hospital in Georgia. They weren't going to let me exercise. I'm eating, I'm eating a ton of food, I'm eating more food than anyone in my family eats, in fact, but no matter how much I eat I'm still hungry. My stomach gets full, so full that it hurts, but my mouth keeps watering for more. It's the weirdest thing. My body doesn't feel sated. But my stomach is stretching. I can't get enough.

And I can't stop running. I can't stop working out.

I take a nap this afternoon. Everything hurts; I'm sad about everything. I ran on the treadmill at the gym this morning— six miles—and then I lifted weights and did ab exercises for another thirty minutes. I showered downstairs in the ladies locker room. Why do they call it that? It isn't a locker room— this is a country club. It's a full-fledged spa lounge, for crying out loud. Everyone in there is older than me. Most of them know me. Most of them pretend like they don't recognize me. A few say hi. Nobody ever reaches out.

After my shower I drive straight to my physician. Her office is on my way home. She weighs me, makes me pee in a cup, mentions that my urine is awfully clear, and am I sure I didn't just drink a ton of water to keep my weight up? I swear I didn't, which is true. I'm standing backwards on the scale (which some doctors require; mine doesn't, but I'm too scared to see the numbers because I know they're slowly going up) while we're having this conversation, while she's weighing me, and I don't know what it says but I know it's up because she's telling me now that I'm doing a great job. Since I decided not to go to the hospital I'm making progress. I'm gaining weight. But I'm a basket case. I'm freaking out. I'm scared.

She tells me, *Make sure you get in some exercise, so that as you gain weight it goes into muscle, not fat.* I think, *If you only knew . . .* but I also think, *Shit, maybe I'm not doing enough. Maybe I need to be lifting more. Maybe I'm not exercising enough for all this new food.*

But I don't say that. I nod instead and make a note to talk to Anne about this next time I see her. Anne is the only one who recognizes that I have a problem with exercise. The physician, maybe that isn't her job. Her job is to treat my underweight condition, whether it's anorexia-induced or otherwise. Her job is to make sure I gain weight, make sure my pulse and blood pressure continue to rise until they're in the normal range, make sure I'm not in immediate medical danger. Anne's the dietitian. I don't know why it's her job to do everything else, but it *is* her job, I guess, because she's good at it. She sees through everything that the other doctors don't see through. My therapist Samuel, I love him, but he won't even talk to me about diet and exercise. He wants to talk about my family, and my ex-boyfriend, and why I'm so sad. And my other therapist, Catherine Lewis, well I only see her in groups and then I have to listen to everyone else talk. So it's Anne who tells me to stop exercising, but I can't.

When I get home I go up to my third-floor bedroom and sprawl magazines all over the floor. I've been working on a scrapbook/journal thing since I started treatment. I've got old letters written to me, new poems I've written myself, photographs, and images from magazines in the mix. Some notes from Tor. I even cut up my meal plans and pasted them in. Today I'm working from a *Playboy* magazine, taping crude cartoons and pictures of naked women, huge breasts, tiny waists into my book, overlapping letters from Christopher and photographs of me that are already fixed onto the pages. At some point I fall asleep. . . .

When I wake up from my nap, I'm cold. I put my orange zip-up hoodie over my halter top and clomp down to the kitchen, looking for Mom. She's in there, cleaning up. She says she came and checked on me, put her hand on my chest to see if I was still breathing. She does this all the time now, whether it's a nap or in the middle of the night. I climb on the counter and grab a bag of cashews out of the cupboard. Mom buys granola ingredients in bulk; her recipe is unbelievably delicious. I've been eating so much granola since I started letting myself taste again, I can't get enough of it. But today I go for the cashews on their own—nothing satisfies me like nuts these days. I crave them constantly—cashews, peanut butter, almonds.

I go into a trance sitting there on the counter, my skinny legs crossed over each other, shoveling handfuls of nuts into my mouth. I can tell that Mom is watching out of the corner of her eye as she's wiping down the soapstone countertops and putting away dishes. I keep eating. Handful. After handful. And more. I don't get full. I can't feel full. I start to cry. I start to cry and then I'm on the floor in Mom's lap and I'm crying about Christopher, I don't know why, and I tell Mom, *I don't know why I'm crying about Christopher, why do I miss Christopher NOW, this is stupid,* and she reminds me of what my doctors, all of them, have said: that once I start to eat again, once there is food back in my body, that's when the real work will begin. That's when the feelings will return. All those months of starvation when I didn't laugh or cry, when I didn't feel anything, when I didn't grieve the loss of Christopher, all that needs to be dealt with now.

I'm a mess of tears when Dad walks in, and he doesn't understand what's going on, why this is so complicated, what the problem is anymore. *Peach is eating,* he thinks. *She's eating and she's gaining weight, so why is she so upset?* I go into a rage. I curse the cashews, the evil cashews that made me cry, I curse my body and the grumbling feeling in my stomach, I curse my mother for being so damn tender and I curse my father for being so out of touch and I grab my running shoes and I'm out the door and in minutes, ahh, relief sets in, in minutes I'm calm again, the rhythmic striking of my feet against the pavement, the immediate relief as if it's needle into vein. I'm happy when I'm running; it's seamless, there's no pain, no confusion, no Christopher or cashews just me and the road and the relief. I run for several miles and then I come back, shower, and eat dinner. Like a normal person. Almost.

# JULY 2001

My mother is standing by me through all of this. She's more than just my mother: She's become my right-hand woman, my best friend, my main supporter. She does not always say the right thing. She does not always know how to handle my mood swings or my battles with mealtime. But she does a few things right. First, she doesn't try to be my therapist. She's there to listen, to hold me and support me, but she doesn't pretend to know better than the professionals. She also admits when she's wrong. And she apologizes. And maybe most important: She's willing to look at her own flaws. Without getting defensive. Without getting angry. She even takes a month off of exercise all together, staying home to monitor and mother me.

I can tell my mom anything. I can push and pull and scream and fight her. I can fall apart in her lap and have a fit about eating a snack. I can binge at night and smoke cigarettes in my bedroom and still, my mom is steady. She doesn't fight back. She doesn't claim to have the answers. She stands by me, she helps me to bed, she tells me she loves me no matter what.

And I need this love, because as I'm beginning to eat and address some of the issues that spurred my eating and exercise disorder, I'm growing deeply depressed. This is pretty common: When the behaviors that a person uses to cope become less available, the pain underneath begins to surface. I am deeply angry, full of violent fantasies, and borderline suicidal. I take a train up to New England to visit friends in July and write in my journal.

July 14, 2001

I have an overwhelming number of suicide and murder fantasies. I still eat a lot at night and less during the day. Fear, food, and exercise take up most of my time. I feel hopeless often. Like there is nothing to live for. I want a boyfriend. That guy at the health food store, even though he smokes. When I masturbate, during my orgasm a violent image overtakes my thoughts: of me pushing over to the ground either Christopher or my father and screaming awful things.

My life is miserable and last night I threatened suicide everywhere; binged; now on a stupid train to Providence they wouldn't let me drive everything is stupid I'm questioning life and relapsing just hate sitting still like this: no calories being burned oh god I want to go home if only I had one.

Eating too many almonds. Doing squats in the bathroom.

An eating disorder is so embarrassing. Why can't I just do it right? Everyone around me so perfect and me on the path to obesity. I dreamt the other night that Mom let her bathrobe fall open in front of the boy I like.

Looking at photos of my tiny arms oh god!!! Why did I stop?? At least then I was numb. At least then I was out of this world that I'm in now and hate so much.

Food is so embarrassing. My ass and fleshy arms are so embarrassing. Last night when Dad asked me what my plan was I said, "to die and kill everyone with me." I sound like the Littleton school shooting killers but instead I'm just a lonely filthy selfish bitch all full of hate and fear. Disgust.

# July 20, 2001

I didn't mean to move to Boston. I meant to take a vacation. My doctors finally let me get out of town for a few days; I'd gained enough weight.

First I went to Providence to visit my high school friend Lindsay. When we were seniors and eighteen years old, we would dress each other up in frilly white petticoats and run barefoot into the snow. I have an old photograph of me in Lindsay's backyard, in a white tank top and petticoat, my blonde hair tangled and long down my back, one arm up in the air, barefoot with snow around my ankles. In the summers we would skinny-dip in Christopher's lake at night. Virginia lakes are warm in the summer, warm enough to linger under water on hot, southern nights. Lindsay and I would swim around the edges to find the muddiest spots, reach down to scoop up handfuls of wet Virginia red clay that made the bottom of the lake, and paint it all over each other's bodies.

On this trip we ran on the beach and put seaweed from the ocean in our hair. After, we got ice cream cones. I thought about weird flavors, like raspberry with chocolate, the kinds of ice cream I don't ordinarily eat. Moose tracks. Whatever.

My next stop was White River Junction, New Hampshire. I went there to see Lily, to stay in her dad's house with the huge garden where they grow snap peas and I don't know what else. I took a walk, we walked, me and Lily and Lily's dad's girlfriend or ex-girlfriend or something. We walked up a big dirt hill and I wore my straw platform sandals. We walked farther than I thought we would.

I arrive in Boston at 5 feet 9 inches and 119 pounds. My leather Longchamp carry-on contains a few halter tops and miniskirts, one pack of American Spirit cigarettes, my cell phone charger, and a journal. Standing outside South Station in platform sandals and red toenail polish, I smoke without making eye contact.

I don't know why I'm here. I took the bus from New Hampshire, and the changeover to catch my train to Virginia was in Boston. But here I still am, standing in a smoker's alley near a T stop behind South Station. Missing my train.

I took the escalator down and found some alley where people were smoking, so I pulled out my cigarettes and now I'm smoking, too. All these men are looking at me. They are, they are all looking at me and I know it's because I've gained enough weight that my face looks normal and my body looks skinny, which means I look like a supermodel and that's why they're looking. I'm thinking about spitting through my cigarette at them. The time in my life I'm the most desired is the time in my life I am least available, and hardly healthy. Sure, I have gained some weight, but mentally I'm not there yet: I can't smile or feel or love myself, let alone love someone else or even lust for them, beyond the violent fantasies that sometimes sweep through me. I can barely finish my cigarette. To my left stands a handsome black college student wearing a short-sleeved button-down, untucked, and carrying a messenger bag. Directly in front of me are two construction workers in hard hats. On my bus from New Hampshire, a German medical student offered me candy. I politely declined by pretending I hadn't heard him; my pen and journal were my cover. I noted that he would age gracefully.

I don't trust any advances because I'm just not myself. I am coming out of a period of starvation, and I know my airbrushed body is a temporary holding space. My flesh has become my battleground: a medium for all my upper-class struggles to manifest through the common rich girl practice of calorie counting. Tedious, and not at all inviting. I wanted to marry the German med student on the bus, but what could I have said to him? *This belly button won't be flat next year. I'll look less fetching in size 12. My designer clothes are hand-me-downs from my adolescent sister. I'm dressed like a hooker to hide the fact that I'm a violent poet.*

Boston in summer isn't much different from Virginia in the summer, weather-wise. I take more risks these days because I'm suicidal. Cramming myself onto a packed green-line T, I am brazen in asking for directions. The car is packed with Red Sox fans headed to Fenway. I know to get off at St. Mary's. I remember the sushi restaurant across the street from Nat's apartment. I grip the pole and watch sweaty gamegoers, with their big bellies and big-bellied sons. They rub their sweat up against my bony arm. I clutch my Longchamp, really stolen from my mother, and clench my toes and jaw.

Ximian isn't brand new, but the company is young enough that spirits are high and Nat's face still wears a freshness and innocence. Today, it turns out, he is in Ottawa. I arrive on his doorstep and am greeted by Matt and Mark, two of Ximian's first employees and Nat's best friends. Someone had called someone to tell someone that I was in Boston instead of headed back home. I last saw Matt and Mark at my graduation party in Charlottesville back in May. I have a photo with Matt from that party: I've got my arm wrenched around his neck like I'm taking him down. My face so skinny, it's a wonder I had the strength to strangle a man, but in fact I had endless energy, spastic, uncontrolled.

I walk up the hard marble stairs, taking in the smell of Boston brownstones. I love the taste in my mouth of that whole city, every building on Beacon Street that same flavor, like musty brick mixed with alcohol. The sound of the door swinging shut behind me. The schlepping sound of my heel coming off the back of my sandal, peeling foot from sweaty shoe, clomping up the stairs.

We sit in the living room of Nat's Brookline apartment, commonly known as the Cave (I'm not exactly sure why). Resided in by Nat, his business partner Mason, and their old friend Tyler. None of whom are home, as I soon learn is a common state at the Cave. I don't feel entitled enough to ask Matt or Mark why they have a key to my brother's pricey apartment, so I recline in the leather chair by the window, and we talk awkwardly: Matt and Mark, myself, and Matt's younger sister Marie: soft blonde curls and bony as me.

Anorexia is a selfish and competitive illness. I don't want to see another skinny girl, and I don't want to think about how I compare to her. I have spent the summer in treatment and am gaining steadily. You still can't locate an ounce of fat on my body outside my breasts, but I'm insecure about how I'll change, and here is Marie, as boldly skeletal as me, in skimpy shorts and high heels. My chewing gum is going stale. I dump my bag on the living room floor.

Tonight turns out to be a premonition of the year to come: taxi rides through Boston, outrageous meals with Matt and Mark, sleeping in Nat's bed while he is out of town. The first of countless evenings clomping up those hard Boston steps to land welcomed and adored in the arms of my brother's life: his apartment, his friends, his food and liquor, his wild imagination. I fall asleep to the laughter and clinking of a party in the condo upstairs, inhabited by Harvard grad students. The first night of many imagining my changing self on the arm of a Harvard man. I feel happy and free, like the typical dream of every typical American girl. When I wake up I go for a run on the path near Nat's apartment and I remember the last time I ran here, less than a year before with Christopher, who I loved so much that same weekend we fucked on the air mattress in Nat's living room. That's the last time Christopher and I had sex; it's actually the last time I had sex at all. The last time I had sex with the man I loved the most was fucking drunk on an air mattress.

Nat charges up the steps the next morning with the same enthusiasm I soon adopt as a critical element of my life in Boston. *Does Mom know you're here? Who's sleeping in Mason's bed? You already went for a run? You're still too skinny. You look better but you're still too skinny. You should call Mom. Come on, let's go have a smoke.*

We climb out the window by the leather chair and onto the balcony. *There's a girl sleeping in Mason's room. That isn't you? Clearly, clearly that isn't you. I'm exhausted. Ottawa was great. We took the red-eye. How did you get here? Let's get some food, we should get some food, you need to eat some food. I started working out. Now I understand why you work out. Man, I feel great! Man, it's great to see you. I love you, Peachie. Is Tyler here?*

Nat's BMW is fast. We pick up Matt and Marie and head for the one and only meal I would ever eat at Leo's Place in Harvard Square: a veggie burger. I sit on the stool at the counter and call US Airways to book a flight home for the next day.

The next day, I call US Airways to change my flight to the following day.

The following day, I call US Airways to change my flight to two days later.

The day after that, Nat goes to work. I walk down to Newbury Street and sit in Trident Booksellers writing postcards and then a letter to my sister at camp. Two hours later I call Nat from a payphone: *I got a job at the Gap. Can I stay with you until I find my own place?*

Something about Boston and my brother's life has taken me in. I don't know why I am so afraid to return to Charlottesville, but it just doesn't feel like a safe place. Each day I've pushed my plane ticket back, thinking I'll be ready to go soon, but when the time comes my panic rises so steadily that I can't bear the thought. I didn't plan on staying in Boston, but at the same time I can't leave. I feel safe here.

Standing on the balcony outside Nat's window, I make the phone call to my mother, asking her to please ship my clothes and other things. I write Victoria a letter, explaining my decision, and send it to her camp address. At twenty-two years old I feel no remorse for not going back to my family, but I'm not prepared for their reactions. Victoria is heartbroken; Mom is angry and feels abandoned. My doctors are concerned: Anne insists that I need to find doctors in Boston if I really am going to stay. Nobody feels that I'm ready to be on my own. But what I know is this: I can recover in Boston. I have to be away from the watchful eyes of everyone who knows I've been sick. I want to rewrite my life, begin again.

I have a love affair with my hometown, I do. Charlottesville, Virginia, is the most erotic place on earth. I love the bricks of the downtown mall; I love the smell of the Mudhouse, my favorite coffee shop. I love the hills between my parents' street and my mom's studio, and I love the feel in my stomach as we rise up and down them in the car. I love the small, feminine mountains that surround Charlottesville: the beautiful Blue Ridge, their calm spirit, their soothing sunsets. I love my old friends, I love the big trees, I love the smell of the streets. But it's an incestuous town. Everyone knows everyone's business, everyone sleeps with everyone's ex-boyfriend, everyone's small business solicits everyone else's small business. In my most resentful phases, we're all just jerking each other off in Charlottesville. And, oh lord, I had to get away.

Boston offers opportunity. New people. People! Actually people, large quantities of them, of many races, of many nationalities, speaking many different languages, wearing many different styles of clothes, and certainly housed in many different size bodies. I can envision a life here of both anonymity and identity. Dating is suddenly a possibility. A career is an option. Bars where I won't run into my parents' friends! Or my first boyfriend, Drew. Or the girl he cheated on me with.

~~~

My long-weekend trip to Rhode Island and New Hampshire became a year in Boston. Recovery is a unique path, individual to each person's particular needs. I did not know that I needed a year in Boston. My doctors, my therapists—they were all concerned when I called to say *I'm not coming home.* I struck a deal with Anne: We exchanged weekly e-mails for nearly that entire year. She kept me on track, kept me moving toward healthy goals, and acted as my go-to person whenever I had a (frequent) relapse or fearful moment. Despite many recommendations, I never hired a local therapist in Boston to treat me. I leaned on Anne, on my mother, and on everything I'd already learned.

## OCTOBER 2001

I don't really know how to build a life for myself here. Especially since September 11, when I briefly considered heading back to Virginia. I still feel pretty scared, but I've just launched myself into freedom and independence, and I'm not quite ready to throw that away.

I take it one day at a time, and one job at a time. I go through three (quickly) before I finally settle into an okay position as an administrative assistant in a cancer hospital. I am paid well, respected, and have my own office. I can walk to work from the gym. I am interacting with people, going out to eat lunch, feeling involved.

Still, most evenings I spend alone, bingeing. And every morning I spend working it off at the gym. I wake up religiously at 5:00 A.M., no matter the weather, and clock a solid workout before walking to work; I also walk home from work at the end of the day. My weight is rising, and I am still terrified, in moments, about my changing body. When will it end? I keep in close touch with Anne, tracking every pound of weight gain, and she continues to encourage me to cut back on exercise, to relax, to buy bigger clothes, to trust my body.

This feeling of "when will it end" is the scariest part of weight gain. I'm about to pass my pre–eating disorder weight, and suddenly I am wearing sizes that are bigger than my pre-anorexic size. I fight this by working out more, walking everywhere, and throwing fits. I binge, I cry, I call my mom in the middle of the night, I vent to Anne in my weekly e-mails to her, I cry again. I stick my finger down my throat once or twice.

I buy all new food, binge on it, and throw it in the garbage. I work out harder. I run an extra mile. An extra mile. An extra mile.

And all the while, all through this ugly, disordered, uncomfortable behavior—I am recovering. I am moving through stages. I am experiencing moments of joy and moments of terror. I am hating my body one hour and loving it the next.

I meet Aaron at my gym. We first introduce ourselves early in the fall, when I still feel thin enough to work out in a bra with no T-shirt over it. He flirts with me once or twice and one morning stops to say, *You exercise too much. Do you even get your period?* I can't believe he has the audacity, the balls, the nerve, but I answer truthfully. *No, I don't. I'm recovering from anorexia, and mind your own business.* He tells me that I am still anorexic, that I am an exercise-induced anorexic, and I think how Anne would agree, and how I'm sneakily managing to gain weight while working out obsessively. I am a little worried now— someone at my gym has been watching me. Aaron expresses more concern and says he wants to work with me to decrease my daily sweat sessions, so we exchange e-mail addresses. And then we make out. Once, twice. He calls inconsistently.

By the end of the month I have my own apartment, in a brownstone near Cleveland Circle. I sometimes walk down to a nearby park before dinner and sit on the swings, wondering if Aaron will call me soon. It is better than thinking about my body, but it's kind of the same, too. Just another thing to obsess over, another reason to decide I'm not good enough.

November 11, 2001

I discovered this evening a blue November dusk in Brookline on the swings near my house. Singing "I am that I am," which implies that I am myself at all. I try to remember that means not my mother, my brother, not Aaron or Christopher, not the earth, the oceans, not the food I eat I am nothing. And swinging the whole time between wholeness and tears (memory of my mother's hands on my body, memory of her carrying me breastless into this world I am so much bigger than her, mourning that) and swinging the whole time thinking I hope someone is recording this!

Last night Nat said about our dinner he wished someone could see it and I thought, like a little girl to her older brother, But Nat I am seeing it! To me you are someone. Am I not someone to you? We were together, I saw, tasted, how well you grilled the salmon. And that was enough someone for me— my brother saw it! He validated it! The food was good. We ate and had coffee afterward, a perfect evening and I was not alone. He saw it. But to him it was as if alone, wasted somehow, with only his sister to see it. Am I not enough?

I have to be honest. I want Aaron to call. I talked about it out loud on the swings with the dark blue sky all around me, blue jeans, long sweater lapping against my calves as I swung. I have to be honest I want him to call. I don't know if I even like him. I want him to like me. Even though I don't know if I like him I want him to call. And I'll feel rejected if he doesn't. He touched me, his hands everywhere even inside me no I will not suck your dick I didn't want to but I left feeling like a disappointment I am not a good lover because I prefer love I guess.

This far into my recovery! My disorder was a longer illness than the months I spent losing weight, and this "recovery" I speak of so much since I began to eat is a recovery from more than starvation. Though the starvation was the symptom. The symptom of my utter rejection of myself. This far into my recovery! And Aaron wants my mouth on him. I haven't seen a penis in a year—he calls it his "cock" and wanted me to kiss it. But I couldn't, I tried to tell him. Why don't men understand? I was all bones. My bones were nearly bending, I imagined holes in them where they began to disintegrate. And he wants my mouth on him! Me thinking the whole time, Can we not just hold hands, go for a walk? That would make me want to kiss him. Leave something to be desired! Please! But so quickly in a bed, naked, and I'm less turned on than when he stands a foot away from me, talking.

But there was one moment. When really in my own despair I flung my naked self backward over his bed, knowing my breasts and belly looked sexy stretched behind, but also to cover my face with my hands, to not see him, to move away from the situation and to recovery into who I am (I am that I am: nothing) and it was then, eyes closed, when he leaned over to retrieve me, to retrieve our (awkward, unsettled, unfinished, not quite) union that I felt myself lusting for him all the way inside me and in that portion of the night I breathed heavily and just remembering it I am breathing heavily again. But something, the part of the brain that's my neuroses, my obsessive, controlling part, worried about everything, consequence, disease. I tried to protect myself and I stopped him again. The animal in me (there is one, I thought maybe she was fully gone but I found her in that moment) wanted to have sex. But numbers came to mind: numbers, blocks, maps, spreadsheets invaded and I came back to awkward, uncertain. Bored, even.

I want a boy to hold my hand, swing with me, buy me ice cream and take me to a movie. I am not here to be 22 and sexual. If he would call and do what he's supposed to do then I would want to sleep with him. Don't men understand how easy it is? Hold my hand. Talk to me. Then I will want you to kiss me, to turn me over in your arms and legs. (Oh—it did feel sweet to smell a body, to share a pillow, a moment.)

He must not like me. None of them do. I ran extra at the gym today. Lately I want to lose weight again—only two pounds. To see if I can do it.

But the truth is all autumn I have been happy alone. I like my rhythm, my routine. I like cooking dinner alone, listening to music, reading David Sedaris books, ignoring my own writing, and indulging in walnuts and cashews.

And if Aaron ever calls? I will have sex with him if he can love me. I promised myself I would not have sex again until I'm married. I promised myself that this summer at the same time I promised myself I'd never get married. At the beach, with Mom. When I was a novelty: so thin still and eating an ice cream cone in the evening; everyone must have envied me! Something so darling about a thin girl eating ice cream. It is much less cute at my weight now. But Aaron will not love me and I will have sex with him anyway if he asks me to, because even though I know better, I still think if I fuck them they will begin to love me. Just like even though I know better, I still think if I'm thin I'll be happier. Truth is—

I am not my strength, not my sex, not my mother. I am not food, not my job, not even my writing. I am only the moment swinging brought: recognition of carelessness, matters not.

When I run far and hard. When I cook. When I swing outside. When I shop at the Copley mall. When I walk down Beacon Street. When I grill salmon with my brother. These are what I am become. I am become a woman. I am stronger than Aaron "suck my cock" and stronger than Nat "I wish someone could see this." I am stronger than my mother "you can pass all your anorexic clothes to me!" I am strong and somehow beautiful without anyone to see it. These moments are valid only in how I view them: only in how they embed themselves in my own heart, my own blue jeans. Size whatever.

## DECEMBER 2001

My room is pink; I painted it myself. The palest shade from the sample strip still stands out in my bedroom. And the walls, they're uneven. Not in height or color, but in length; it's a five-walled room, an uneven shape. I've put the bed in a crook where the walls make a cozy, circular curve. Aaron doesn't say anything about the room. He doesn't say anything except *Come here, baby,* which makes me laugh. At him. We climb in bed together, Christmas Eve, me and the man I'm about to lose my second virginity to. That's how I think about it—a second slicing of the seal. In many ways this second time means so much more than the first, the first time seven years ago with Drew on a bathroom floor somewhere, in some building I do remember but wish I didn't. Wish I couldn't describe how the basement computer lab smelled, but I do remember: I remember the bathroom was around a corner, how we made out there, and how one day it happened—I was no longer a little girl—but it was so unconscious, so unplanned, totally unsymbolic, uncelebrated, empty.

This time I know it's going to happen, and I know what it means. It means I'm choosing life, welcoming myself as a woman back into the world, opening myself to feeling both pleasure and pain, the potential for heartache, opening to the possibility of attachment: man to woman, woman to man, heart to heart but—

In this case nothing so special happens. Aaron and I screw; I don't pay attention to the details, except that he sweats and then says, *It's not like I do this all that often,* which is reassuring, considering I haven't done it in over a year and the last time was with Christopher, who I loved and who loved me and I know it was true and this time I know I'm doing it to get back to the other side, to the land of the living and when it's over we talk about pickles and bacon, he likes them, I'm conscious of my body it's covered and he falls asleep I can't believe it I'm smiling, smirking really wow—back on the other side.

I'm staying in Boston for the holidays this year. I'm not ready to go back to Charlottesville. I want to forget every memory from childhood, forget all the Christmases when we waited at the top of the tall stairs for Dad to give the "all clear" sign, the sign that Santa had come, that there were gifts under the tree, on the couches and leather lounge chairs, that there were stockings laid across the ottoman, one for each child, and we would open them in a fury and compare new toys and clothes, later lipsticks and jewelry. I want to forget Christmas brunch, the smoked salmon and omelets, the toasted bagels, the hot cocoa, the slippers on the soft kitchen floor, the fresh-squeezed orange juice from the old fruit squeezer, the one that looked like a tin man in a pointy hat. I want to forget the Christmas before, when our relatives from France were visiting and we laughed and went to the movies and I drank a big Diet Coke. I want to forget the long run I took on Christmas morning and how earlier that week I'd tried to throw up the cookie dough I'd eaten and couldn't, couldn't get it out of me, and I want to forget that I have a family, a big one, one that loves me and wants me to be well. I want to forget the good and the bad, the all of it, the photo taking and celebrating. I want to take just two days off work and spend them with Nat, spend them going for runs around Brookline, around the reservoir near my apartment, passing the tall, lean men, passing the college girls jogging together. I want to shop downtown in Boston and watch other families reunite for the season, watch old high school friends run into each other at the mall. I want to talk to my own family as quickly as possible, get it over with and be on the other side.

I cook for him, not Aaron but Nat, on Christmas Eve. I make risotto and we have a salad. We run across the street afterward so Nat can buy cigarettes, and it's cold but I sit in a skirt, bare legs, on the curb across the street from the brownstone where I live. After dinner Nat gives me a pep talk, one that should be memorable but again I don't really pay attention to the details, only that his face is fierce with love as it sometimes is these days, often is, as he helps pull me from despair. I don't know if I tell him Aaron is coming over later, I don't know if he would care, or what he would say, but he goes home without me, Nat does, back to his own apartment a couple of miles away.

Aaron doesn't arrive with wine or flowers. But he is wearing a hat, and I am wearing green Adidas sneakers, and I haven't shaved my legs because I don't care that much, but I know what's going to happen. When he kisses near my ankle I think, *I am probably the only girl he's been with who hasn't shaved her legs,* but I'm so fair and my leg hair is white, so in all likelihood he doesn't notice; he's just thinking about what comes higher up my leg and how quickly he can get there and get out.

He falls asleep, though he doesn't mean to. I listen to him breathe and can't fall asleep myself, so I go to the kitchen in my green terrycloth robe, not Christmas green but spring green, like Easter, and tuck my hair behind my ears, making myself a peanut butter sandwich on raisin bread. Then I do fall asleep, next to him, a man, in my bed, on Christmas Eve. He wakes up at 2:00 A.M. and leaves my house, kisses my mouth, says, *I'll call you tomorrow,* and I wonder immediately why he says that. He won't. And then he says *Merry Christmas,* and I say *You're Jewish* and he says *So?* And I latch the door behind him.

In the morning I run far enough to make my legs hurt, an extra mile, maybe two. I make myself a special breakfast, as special as it can be, alone, twenty-two years old in an empty apartment in Brookline, winter in Boston, my cheeks pink from my run. Later, when I think Nat might be awake, I take the T to his apartment. We drive with his friends to a Jewish deli, the only place open on Christmas Day serving real food, and I hesitate over towering sandwiches and fat galore. Ultimately and joyously I choose a corned beef sandwich on rye, and I eat it (although it confuses me that people eat this much meat and bread) and drink a Dr. Brown's black cherry soda. I remember doing this with my father at the Carnegie Deli in New York and think, *I'm doing this for you, Dad,* even though I'm so far away, and far away on purpose.

Nat and I simulate Christmas by opening the gifts Mom has sent. And it is sad, the whole affair, and unsatisfying, and I go back to my own apartment in the early evening; I don't know why I don't stay with Nat, stay with my family, but that I'm a loner and I'm lonely and I probably want to binge, and so I do. I go back alone, in the dark, and I eat too much peanut butter and too much chocolate and I get in bed and I think about what it felt like last night, and did it feel good? And I don't even know.

I don't remember the rest of the night, or the next few days, but I know Aaron did not call until it had been long enough for me to tell myself to get over him. I had re-lost my virginity and I was back on the other side, the side of the living, but I could not stop running too far in the mornings . . . and hurting my legs.

## FEBRUARY 19, 2002

I'm sitting in a cozy, dark, wooden restaurant somewhere in downtown Boston with another writer, a girl I met at a poetry reading. I want to leave. I feel distracted and uncomfortable. It's snowing outside, it's such a beautiful night, but I feel awkward and not willing to open up and make friends. I tell her anyway that I'm in recovery from an exercise compulsion. I tell her because I'm honest, despite not wanting to be her friend or wanting to sit here at all. She orders wine; I don't want any. I'm explaining that I'm learning how to exercise less, to moderate my workouts, to slowly wean off of exercising. She says quickly, *I wish I had that problem!*

I don't know then how to guide the conversation smoothly. I feel violated, angry, confused. I try to explain why it's possible to exercise too much, that, in fact, a lot of women do it, that it's a real illness. But I think I come across sounding desperate and confused. Which, of course, I am.

## SPRING 2002

My year in Boston continues. I improve. My work with Anne progresses. I begin to accept my body as my weight gain steadily slows. I don't have to buy new clothes every two weeks anymore. I don't feel so afraid of what I am eating. I still binge sometimes and I still work out religiously, but I have made some progress in acceptance. I can see, more realistically, how my body compares to other women's bodies. I see my body more for what it is: a sturdy, healthy frame, an excellent tool for getting things done, for experiencing pleasure.

Aaron and I fall into a noncommittal pattern of occasional sex and infrequent telephone calls. I care, but I don't care that much. I care more about my recovery. I've read several books about eating disorders and decided that I'd be an excellent advocate for recovery. I want now, I genuinely want, a full recovery, a full life, a healthy relationship with my body. I can see now, with a bit more perspective, the dangerous position I put myself in and how much work is really required to get better. I can understand now, as my doctors told me, how a full recovery really could take ten years.

I speak strongly about body acceptance. I write letters to companies that portray women's bodies disrespectfully in ads, or that confuse messages of food and guilt. I vehemently educate my mother on all the horrible things she did to instill an eating disorder in me: criticize her body in front of me, talk about weight in an insensitive manner, cut her cookie in half instead of eating the whole thing. She listens. That's what's amazing about my mother: She's impossible to hate, even when she screws up, because she listens and then says *I'm sorry*. And she means it.

Despite my real efforts to accept my body, at this point I still struggle with it. I secretly think that I want to accept my body but keep it reasonably small. I see that this is hypocritical, but it's what I want anyway. So I talk to everyone about body acceptance but I work out obsessively because I'm scared of gaining more weight. I'm confused, but at least I know it.

What I don't know yet, but am about to find out, is that my excessive exercise is not only keeping a full recovery at bay, but slowly working my body to a pulp. I'm about to discover the woes of overuse injuries.

# MAY 9, 2002

The yoga teacher is late. I'm standing at the back of the room and all I can think about is how my ass looks in these spandex capris that I've been wearing since I was skinny and am still wearing, despite how much weight I've gained, which is about thirty pounds, and I'm pretty self-conscious. I keep turning my head, looking for Aaron. I'm at the health club where we met and he could be here. And then there he is, back on the floor talking to a woman right by the door to the studio room where I'm waiting with everyone else for the yoga teacher to arrive. I try to turn, contort my body to show him a better angle, but I don't know if he even sees me or knows I'm in the room.

It's hard to be calm in the yoga class after seeing Aaron. We've been on and off since we met in October, and my body has changed. I'm working out twice most days now, again; I was at the gym this morning before work and now I'm sweating through yoga after work, all of this to keep my weight gain in check. Despite these efforts, my body continues to grow. I guess it wants to.

I get off the T after yoga, the D line at Beaconsfield, and I walk by the kids playing softball and I'm smiling, I don't know why, all the way to my doorstep. Nobody is home. Nobody calls me. I make a big salad for dinner and write for a while at my laptop on the kitchen table. Afterward I go for a run around the reservoir: my third workout of the day.

I keep in touch with Anne in our weekly e-mails, still. She doesn't know, exactly, that I'm working out this much. I am happier; I'm more comfortable with food. I stress this in my messages to her, but I do occasionally reveal that I can't let go of my workouts. I can't let them go, and I'm not happy without them. I'm considering really trying to take a full week off my workouts. I mention this to Anne sometimes and she supports the idea, suggesting an even longer break, but I think starting with a week is all that I can offer just yet.

# MAY 14, 2002

I'm in the elevator with my boss. I feel pretty good; it's spring and my new white Banana Republic skirt looks sharp with a slim-fitting pinstripe button-down. I'm holding a handful of files and we're talking about what to order for the next lunch meeting, both of us in good moods. I shift a little in my heels. The elevator makes a weird noise and lurches and we look at each other, my eyes must be wide, but then it eases back to normalcy and we land on our floor safely and laugh. My boss goes into his office after I slip into mine, next door, and close the door most of the way.

It's a normal day at work. I have a stack of papers I haven't even looked at sitting on my desk and several meetings to arrange, and I need to check the voice mail—but nothing time-sensitive that I can't finish by the end of the day, and I'm happy with spring in the air. I grab a folder with slides and let my boss know I'm running over to the neighboring hospital's photo lab to finish up the order for the project we're working on. My boss is a department head at Boston's premier cancer hospital, and he has to give a big talk next week that I'm not behind in preparing, thank goodness. I walk by the cafeteria on my way out, smile at the guy behind the counter who flirts with me, and skip up the stairs to the first floor and out onto a busy, sunny Boston sidewalk.

At some point I notice my right shoulder aches. I switch the folder I'm carrying over to the left side and circle my right arm around a bit, moving my shoulder backward and forward, in and out of socket. Strange. It aches. When I get back to my desk I take an ibuprofen and finish up the day.

I get off the T several stops early and walk the rest of the way home, thinking about what to make for dinner. It will be salad. It's been salad a lot lately—a big salad with tuna fish, some almonds, maybe, tomatoes and orange peppers. Part of why I feel so good lately is that I'm back in control with food. I'm working out multiple times a day and haven't let myself binge in weeks. I feel like I've really nailed it, because I'm eating what I want to during the day, even getting milk shakes in the food court as an afternoon snack. But healthy dinners and no bingeing are helping my clothes fit better. I still don't weigh myself; I haven't since the fall. Anne encourages me not to read my weight until I'm recovered enough to not care what it says, and I wonder if that will ever happen. At this point, I just don't want to know.

The next morning, I notice something is definitely wrong with my shoulder. At the gym I have to modify my strength work, which frustrates me. I keep trying to identify how I might have hurt it, and the only thing I can think of is all the arm-balancing poses in yoga class. I hate thinking I'm not strong enough to take it, that something is wrong with my body. But I decide to replace my evening yoga class with cycling and figure that probably burns more calories anyway, so I get over it.

# JUNE 2002

In June I go home for my birthday. Mom and I take five nights alone together at the Sanderling Inn on the Outer Banks of North Carolina. We go for runs on the beach in the morning, or I go to the resort's gym to ride the bike while Mom stretches on our balcony. At night we cook together in the little kitchenette and I laugh nervously and excitedly to see how much oil Mom puts on our pasta salad. I eat it, and it tastes good. I like it; I'm still excited by food, more excited by food than anything else. We get ice cream cones on the boardwalk like we did last year when I was so much thinner, and remembering that makes me sad, makes me long for length—that enviable pair of legs that strolled in the sunshine just one year ago. But I know life is better now, and I focus on my strength and athleticism.

We drive back to Charlottesville together, stopping at a fruit stand and talking about how much we love being together. When we pull into the driveway, I can see Daddy and Tor bounding around in the kitchen through the windows. Tor has bought me so many goofy birthday presents, the kind of stuff I love: matching underwear for both of us, matching red tube tops, matching skirts. I love having a sister, and mine is so beautiful right now. I think I was so awkward at her age, but she is lovely, tan, happy, all smiles. Nat joins us in Charlottesville that afternoon, and we all go for dinner at the country club. There are photos from that evening: me in black with the little birthday cake the club offers sitting in front of me, one candle lit. Happy family, I feel. Happy Peach.

Two days later, Nat and I drive my truck back up to Boston. I've decided I know the city well enough now to have a car up there. It will help with groceries, and with weekend summer getaways. I want to go to the Cape; I haven't been there since I was a kid. I want to drive to the mall in Newton. I want to visit my friends in nearby states. So we load up an old armoire in the back, which I've also decided I want with me in Boston, and head north. Nat drives. I read out loud from José Saramago's *Blindness.* I'm anxious that I won't be working out today but am telling myself everything Anne tells me: namely, that you can't change your body in a day. It sort of works, but I start fidgeting as much as possible, stomping my feet and flailing my arms to burn calories. Nat thinks it's funny, so we do it together. I justify that I just want to *move,* you know, uncomfortable in the car, but probably my brother knows what I'm really thinking.

We get lost at some point on the drive, which makes it longer, and at another point we stop for McDonald's and get french fries, which make us both feel sick. I take a lot of pictures out the window, and we laugh most of the way up. I'm happy the whole drive with Nat, but in my first week back in Boston I decide I'm moving back home to Charlottesville. My week vacation instilled so much confidence in me. I went for a visit with Anne while I was home, and she was so proud of me—so happy to see me with full hips and a smile on my face. Look what I've done! Look at the weight I've gained! I supported myself for a whole year in a city without my parents' help, I managed an entire office for an important doctor, I brought myself from danger of dying into an exuberant, nearly recovered state. And I dated!

My boss takes the news okay, but the girl in human resources tells me that my supervisor said I was the best assistant they ever had. I'm offered a promotion and a raise to stay, but I feel

I have bigger fish to fry, though I don't know what yet. I think I want to write a book. I think I want to work in eating disorder outreach. And, I decide with clarity, I need to return home to finish the work I started. I ran away to Boston nearly a year ago and left a lot of loose ends back home.

# JULY 19, 2002

Before moving back home, I fly to Los Angeles to visit Casey. When I step off the plane she says, *You're thinner than I thought you'd be!* And then, *I want your bag! Can I carry it?* It's my mother's Louis Vuitton that I coveted for years and finally stole; after all, she never carries it anymore. I think I saw Madonna carrying the same bag in a magazine.

My first night in Los Angeles, Casey and I go for dinner at a Vietnamese restaurant. We both get noodle dishes and drinks—she's into martinis, extra dirty, and I go for my usual summer favorite: gin and tonic. I feel like we're best friends again, talking easily, appreciating our always differing opinions on every topic from how to raise children to politics to bodies and fashion. The next morning we go shopping and then to the gym. I wear my workout clothes to the mall, and she's embarrassed by it and asks me to put on the skirt I just bought in J. Crew. *No,* I tell her, *I want to wear it tonight when we go out.*

That night I'm tired before we've even left the house. I don't drink much; I never have, as my body can't really handle it. We have dinner with Casey's boyfriend and she drinks two martinis, then we go to a party where everyone has some wine, and then onto a bar, some sort of tropically themed outdoor place that would be fun if I had more energy or was friends with anyone there. But I'm flying back to Boston in the morning, so I figure I can last the night. Someone orders me a drink, and I sip it and then go get some water by the bathrooms. Casey is still drinking, and I marvel at her tolerance.

We decide to go home. We get in her car. She's driving. I don't remember if I ask whether she's okay to drive. I remember pulling out. I remember an intersection. I remember seeing the headlights and grill of a big truck heading for me, the passenger side of the car, and I know that Casey let go of the wheel and grabbed for me, let go of the wheel and hugged me, screamed something, maybe my name.

Now everything is still and I can't hear or see very well, but someone is looking at me. They want to help me out of the car. I am in a car? I reach for a handle. They are telling me I can't get out that way. They are telling me the door doesn't work, but I don't register this. I am in a car? Who are the people looking at me? Now I am somehow in the grass. *Do you want to go to the hospital?* I stare. *Do you want to go to the hospital?* I stare. I am thinking, *The hospital? Why am I in the grass? Why do I need to go to the hospital?* And then I am able to know at least that I am scared, so yes, I want to go to the hospital. In college once I had a panic attack and I went to the hospital. I like doctors. I always feel safe with doctors. I say, *Yes, I want to go to the hospital,* and Casey laughs and says I don't need to. Casey takes my phone from my bag and calls her boyfriend.

I'm in the ambulance. They ask me if I know where I am and I say no, but I can tell them my name and my birth date and I can tell them my address in Boston. They tell me I am in Los Angeles and then I remember why I came here, that I have a friend here, but it takes a while longer until I can remember what happened this evening.

When I get to the hospital the nurse takes all my clothes off and rolls me on a stretcher to the radiology department for a CT scan. I tell the tech, *I work in a hospital, too, in Boston.* They roll me back into the room where I was with the first nurse. She comes in to check on me. I ask where my friend is, and I'm thinking she was probably arrested. I'm thinking they probably took a breathalyzer and she is probably in jail. I think to myself, *This will bring us closer than ever.* But the nurse tells me she's waiting outside for me, and several hours later, when the CT scan comes back normal and the nurse tells me I have a concussion but should be okay, just to please monitor it, and I'm released, I walk outside and meet Casey and she says, *I knew you'd be okay. I knew you were just being dramatic, Peach.*

When I land in Boston I leave her a message to say I made it safely home. I take three days off work, and it takes ten days for the bump on my head to disappear and the cuts on my hands to fade. I get a gentle, relaxing massage, sleep a lot, and cry. Aaron promises to bring dinner by one night but never calls when he says he will.

# AUGUST 15, 2002

By the time I return to work, my days in Boston are truly numbered. Nat throws a fabulous dinner party one hot night, after I give a poetry reading at WordsWorth Books in Harvard Square. We went down there a few nights earlier to see the poster in the window—it's my face! My face, blown up huge on a poster, and I remember jumping up and down and whooping in the streets of the square with Nat and his friends, yelling at cars driving by, *Hey, that's ME up there!* The reading goes well, I feel dazzling lately, and Nat's dinner party is decadent as always. Afterward we hit the bars in Cambridge, and I dance with Tyler at the Good Life. Everyone crashes at the Cave that night, me in the guest room, and the next morning I wash the dishes, throw out all the cigarette butts, and vacuum the carpets before anyone else wakes up. I grab a coffee from Dunkin' Donuts across the street and walk back to Nat's apartment to sit on the stoop and call Mom on my cell. I tell her the party felt like the first of my good-byes, and we talk about how in the moment you're getting ready to leave somewhere, it suddenly seems like it has so much to offer. But I'm adamant: It's time to come back home.

The week Aaron and I have a good-bye dinner, I finally commit myself to taking seven full days off of exercise. Anne and I have been working on this in our e-mail sessions, and she's still concerned that I'm doing too much. I'm scared to take a week off, but I'm in a phase where I want to do what I'm afraid of. Recovery is still exciting and fun. I'm replacing working out with social dates in the evenings and drinking coffee in the mornings. I decide I like having a little more time to sleep in, so I start eating breakfast at home before I take the T to work, which reminds me of being a little kid and eating at the table with Nat before school.

Today my hair is down. I'm working late most nights this week to finish up every last loose end for the new assistant who's taking my place. Plus, the work focus is helping me stay away from the gym. Aaron is supposed to pick me up at 7:30, so I stay at work until then. My boss walks by my office around 7:00 and looks curiously at me as he waves good-bye. It's the first time he's ever left before me.

Aaron picks me up in front of the hospital where I work, and we go for casual food somewhere in Brookline. He suggests I be a cheap date and order the $5 hamburger special, and I threaten him with all the stories I'll tell when I finally write a book. *I'm not going to change your name,* I say. Then I tell him, *Anyway, I'm paying.* He says that he has a feeling this isn't the last we'll see of each other, and I think about that when I get home later that night, dropped off outside my brownstone with only a little kiss on the corner of my mouth. It's been less than a year since I met Aaron, and we've had sex, yes, and it's been fun, yes, and he seems to care about me but not necessarily enough to keep in touch, so I decide I doubt him, what he's said about us not seeing the last of each other. And I pack my things that weekend and get ready to move back down south.

# LATE AUGUST 2002

Nat helps me pack up a U-Haul and hugs me good-bye, and I drive by myself in that clunking truck down I–95, through New York City, around D.C., and into Charlottesville. I arrive at midnight. My family is at the beach, so I let myself into their big house and sleep in my parents' bed until they return home. I'm going to be living in a cottage they own, just half a mile away. It's adorable! I've fantasized about living there my whole life.

When I wake up in the morning, I throw a bike in the back of the U-Haul with all my stuff and head over to the little cottage, my new home. I'm pretty impressed with how I single-handedly unload the whole thing, even that monstrous armoire I brought up to Boston just two months ago. When I'm finished I drop the truck off in the U-Haul parking lot and climb on the bike I brought with me to ride back home.

Settling into Charlottesville is fun. Dinner with Mom and Dad and Tor every night! Good food! Dance classes at Studio 206, shopping, sunning myself at the pool. I work out every morning and still sometimes in the afternoons, too. I hang out with my high school friend Jane and Mom's assistant at the Studio, Bethany, who I'm becoming friends with, but mostly I spend time enjoying setting up my own home, planning the garden I never end up planting, and taking a break from work.

# EARLY SEPTEMBER

I fly back up to Boston for a weekend with my mother to bring my truck home. We left it in the hands of a friend, but now I need it back. In the meantime, the shoulder injury that I felt first when I was living in Boston has returned and intensified and I've developed sciatica. Again. This isn't my first episode—I've had it before, a couple of different times, over the last few years of my regular running. We stay with Nat in his apartment. I hang out, mostly, while Mom helps him shop for things. When we go together to Bed Bath and Beyond, my cell phone rings; it's Aaron. Mom answers and he says, *Hey, baby,* thinking it's me. We're in the same shopping center where Nat's office and Aaron's health club are located, so he runs down and meets us in the parking lot for a quick hug. Seeing Aaron makes me miss him. He shows me the watch he bought in Amsterdam, we kiss good-bye, and I keep thinking, *Maybe he'll call, tell me he's madly in love with me.* But by our last night in Boston I'm too distracted to think about Aaron. I can't stop crying because of the pain in my shoulder, now running down my arm. I can't move my arm overhead. Mom puts me in the bath, but it doesn't help. She chastises me for overexercising, which I deny. *You push yourself too hard, Peach,* she tells me. *This is your body responding. Please listen to it.*

Mom has to drive the whole way home because I can't shift gears with my shoulder the way it is. In fact, I can't move my right arm at all. I have to move it with my left arm. And I have to change sitting positions every minute or so, the sciatic pain running down my right leg. I'm loaded up with ibuprofen, but it doesn't seem to be helping much.

We stop at a motel somewhere, and Mom and I go to use the gym. I run on the treadmill, and while I'm moving the stiffness in my leg loosens, but I have to be careful about moving my arm. It makes the run almost impossible, and I feel defeated.

When we get back home, I see a sports medicine specialist, at UVa's hospital. He tells me almost nothing, insists I need an MRI. But I can't get an MRI. I don't have health insurance. And I can't get health insurance. I have a history of anorexia. It's in my medical records.

There's not much I can do. Anne continues to recommend rest, rest, rest. My mom recommends bodywork: gentle massages, easeful stretching, and warm baths. I take a lot of ibuprofen, apply ice twice a day to every corner of my body, and whimper through the nights.

## SEPTEMBER 16, 2002

I e-mail Aaron once in September, shortly after I see him on that trip to retrieve my truck. I tell him I want to become a personal trainer and I need his advice on choosing a certification program. He never responds, so I make my own decision and begin studying for the exam.

Casey calls one night when I'm at my parents' house, curled up in Mom's little lounge room, reading my PT manual and trying to comprehend all the science of slow and fast twitch muscles. I can understand that well enough, but when I get to the chapter on how the body metabolizes sugar I'm completely lost, even with the diagrams. Especially with the diagrams.

We talk very carefully. It's our first conversation since the car accident. She doesn't mention that, but I tell her what's going on in my life: *I'm studying to be a personal trainer. I'm working at Mom's studio, getting used to life in C'ville again.* I have no idea what she tells me, but it's clear that she doesn't seem interested or impressed with my pursuits. We hang up. I feel chilly and go downstairs for a snack.

## OCTOBER 1, 2002

I take a job as a secretary in the OR Department of UVa's hospital. I walk there early every morning; I have to be at my desk by 7:00 A.M. Sometimes I see friends of my parents out walking their dogs, getting their exercise in before work. I hate this job. I can't relate to anyone here, and my coworkers make fun of me for how quickly I finish projects. *Look who's gonna be the next manager,* they say. Most of the day I type e-mails to friends, because every time I ask my supervisor for a new project she acts like I'm putting her out. After work I go to the gym. My pain has eased a bit, but I have to be careful: It returns sometimes without warning, and when it does, it's unbearable. But not exercising is more unbearable, and often the endorphins kick in early enough that I can get through my workout with more exhilaration than pain, and oh, I need that rush, I need that because my life is so pathetic.

My membership at the UVa fitness center is the best perk of my job. I walk home in the evenings, eat dinner alone, call Mom crying, and go to sleep. It's the worst job I've ever had, I decide, certainly worse than selling cotton candy on the downtown mall Friday nights in high school, and so one day I just don't go back.

I call Aaron to tell him I had a job for three weeks. We haven't talked since that day at Bed Bath and Beyond, but I'm in high spirits when I call, mainly because during my brief tenure at the hospital, a coworker with a fake gold tooth kept asking me out. I leave Aaron a flirty message on my way to the gym, and he calls me back almost immediately, suggesting we meet up for a weekend of sex sometime soon. I'm ecstatic.

Mom is compassionate about my decision to quit; she thinks I need some time to decompress and not worry about making a living, so I strike a deal with my parents that I can live rent-free in the cottage for one year. I'll make enough working at Mom's studio to pay for everything else, and once I finish my personal trainer certification, I'll have more options. I join Anne's body image group and refocus my efforts on recovery.

## OCTOBER 17, 2002

The first night in group I'm wearing a new long-sleeve T-shirt, a designer brand, so the cotton is exceptionally soft, and it's a slim-fit with a royal-looking emblem, in gray, in the center of the chest. With my J. Crew jeans. And clogs. Lately I'm wearing my hair down and wavy, cut straight across the bottom, no layers. No makeup.

I like Charlotte the second she walks in. She's comfortable casual, gray sweatpants and a colorful polka-dot fleece. Cute sneakers. She curls up on the couch, sitting cross-legged in the corner, bright blonde hair, southern smile.

I'm in group therapy, after my year in Boston, after my significant weight gain. I don't look sick anymore. My behaviors are still somewhat disordered but I feel very recovered compared to when I first walked into Anne's office, so underweight and scared. I remember that on that first day Anne told me I wasn't well enough to join one of her groups, that I wouldn't be well enough to join one of her groups until I had gained back enough weight to handle the emotional work. I didn't understand that then, but it's over a year later and now I do understand, because I have gained enough weight, plenty of weight, but there is so much pain in my heart that hasn't gone away. There is so much confusion about my body and food that still needs to be resolved.

Anne's office is in her house, so her group meets in the living room. All the girls are different sizes—two are clearly anorexic, another is heavier than me, a few of us look generally healthy but in this setting you can tell we're all a little disturbed. Anxious glances. Clutching tea cups. Fiddling with pens, or twirling hair. I feel nervous when I speak, but later people tell me they admire my ability to talk about my feelings articulately, and with so much confidence. At the end of the meeting we're supposed to write (on pieces of paper that only Anne will see) about what it felt like to be in a room with all these other young women struggling in similar ways. I write, *I like Charlotte. I know we'll be friends.*

Soon my group is my social life. The anxious twirling and clutching subside a bit. We meet sometimes for dinner out (which turns into a big mistake for the girls who are still not comfortable eating in public, or eating at all), and eventually a few of us become especially close.

## NOVEMBER 2, 2002

Charlotte hosts a get-together at her house one night. I arrive a little late since I had to sub a class at Mom's studio. We all sit around openly gabbing about our eating disorders, our ex-boyfriends, our families. Charlotte's roommate Claire is sitting on the couch reading and probably listening, I think, probably thinking we all sound crazy, how brazenly we're saying things like *My parents had an affair* or *I made myself throw up three times last week* or *I was raped in a fraternity house,* but these are the conversations that become the foundation of our friendships. We need each other. We need a place to say those things out loud. To be heard.

I love Charlotte's house. I love her neighborhood. I love getting to know Charlotte, taking long walks downtown as fall becomes winter, drinking hot chocolate in cafes in our sweatpants, writing supportive e-mails to each other during the day when we doubt something about what we ate, or didn't eat, or whether we're working out. At night we go to Arch's for frozen yogurt and order gooey chocolate brownie toppings on our desserts. Lots of times Andrea—another girl from the group—joins us with her boyfriend Jonathan. Having a boyfriend seems so far away! I marvel at Andrea's ability to be both in treatment and in a relationship. One night we're supposed to bring a support person to group. Almost all of us bring our mothers, but Andrea brings Jonathan. My eating disorder and my mother are still my primary relationships, even though I've been through a year of Aaron on and off, and even though I feel well enough to function normally in most settings.

But not all settings. After a year of keeping a busy job in Boston, I'm not working in Charlottesville, not really. I've regressed a bit from feeling confident enough to manage my own life in a busy city. In Charlottesville, depression is setting in.

I am helping Mom out at her studio, folding towels, answering phone calls, guiding new students toward appropriate classes. But I'm making my own hours, without which arrangement I probably could not work. My necessity to have complete control over so many details of my life is still fairly consuming: I need to clean my house every day. I need to fold every T-shirt the way I learned in the boutique where I used to work. I need to be alone every morning, to eat breakfast alone and to work out alone. And I need this to happen in my own timing: If I want to sleep a little later one day, I need that to be okay. I need to be alone before bed, too, to have my nighttime snack alone, to sleep alone. A job would upset my routine because it would be an imposition on my priorities. Mom lets me work when I want to. I help out on days when I have energy and hide out in my little cottage on days when I'm depressed, renting movies and baking cookies. I am able, sometimes, to meet friends for lunch and Charlotte for frozen yogurt at night. I am able, sometimes, to laugh at the movies and run into old friends downtown and be happy to see them.

But the longer I'm home—now that I have weight back on my body, now that the symptoms of my disorder are fading, now that I look normal again—the more depressed I feel. Worse than before. All the pain I ran from. All the pain I hid with my eating disorder. Is now in the forefront. I have to deal with it. I cry. I sleep. I binge on cookies, and cookies and peanut butter, and peanut butter and soy milk, and soy milk and cookies again. I run, as much as I can, all over town. I dance in classes at my mom's studio. As much as I can. I go to yoga as often as I can, when my shoulder can take it. And

I go to therapy. I sit in Samuel's office, and I cry. About my parents. Who now live together again, who have lived together since I started treatment, but who I'm still not sure are happy. And I never really understood what happened with them anyway. Never found out why they separated. Never had any of my suspicions confirmed. And never felt convinced that they belonged together to begin with, my parents, and that therefore I belonged on this planet to begin with myself.

So I make my bed meticulously. I don't let anyone into my house. I leave my shoes at the door and plump the pillows on my couch and dust my laptop and arrange the colorful bowls in my cupboard and eat only organic food, even when I binge, except when I go to Arch's with Charlotte. And sometimes, when I'm with Charlotte, I feel happy. And sometimes, in those moments, I can see outside of the depression; I can even feel the purpose of the depression. To feel the pain I avoided. I came back to Virginia, in part, to deal with what I ran away from when I moved to Boston: my family life, my old fears, myself. So I'm slowly dealing with it, with the help of Samuel, and Anne, and Charlotte, and my mom. And slowly, slowly, I trust this depression will fade. Despite periods of hopelessness, I do believe in myself. I do trust myself. And I will move forward.

# DECEMBER 4, 2002

It's an overcast Wednesday morning, and I'm driving through Charlottesville to take my proctored personal trainer certification test at Sylvan Learning Center. I've never been here before. I pull into the parking lot and sit in my truck for a few minutes, looking over my note cards, quizzing myself on a few kinesiology terms (sagittal, frontal, horizontal). I'm not really worried about passing; I've taken a few home tests and have done pretty well. In fact, I'm assuming I'll pass. I've already lined up a client starting after Christmas. Through the studio Mom found someone who wants personal training at her home gym a few times a week.

I'm nervous and excited to train clients. My own relationship with exercise is still imperfect. I think I take better care of myself now. I recognize that I'm still dependent on working out, that I'm still prone to injury, and that I still don't always do what my body says, but I am *listening* to it. I hear it loud and clear, in fact. And I've learned, through working with Anne and studying for this exam, why all the overtraining doesn't do me any good. I'm ready to make changes, I think. And I am making some. But I know in my heart that I'm not quite there yet, not 100%.

I wonder: Will training clients help me recover, or will it trigger me to work out more? Will focusing on someone else's body help me forget about my own, or will it push me into competitive behavior and self-doubt? What will my clients think of my body? Do I look like a personal trainer? What should a personal trainer look like? I'm not skinny; I'm actually kind of curvy. I am bigger now than I was before my eating disorder. But I like my body, at least sort of. I do doubt it sometimes, but

I'm working on acceptance and that work pays off. I'm telling myself that it doesn't matter what my clients think my body looks like—I'm going to be there to educate them on balanced, healthy exercise. I'm there to explain how the body works and to make recommendations for them. My work as a trainer is not going to be about being skinny or losing weight; it's going to be about feeling good in your body and finding activities you enjoy. I've decided this already. I'm still teaching it to myself.

# JANUARY 7, 2003

I go to Wet Seal to buy jeans—sex jeans. I'm hot, even if I've never been this fat. Is it fat? Am I fat? What does fat mean? Everything is fat compared to how I used to be. I feel fat every day, and I compare my body to everyone else's, and it always looks bigger. I have no idea if it really is, but that's how it looks. I think I start to convince people that I am actually fat, and maybe I am, because they treat me that way now. At least this is how I see it.

They are ass-tight, the jeans I buy; they paint down my leg like nylons. If I wear them with a boot, a boot with a heel. If I wear them with a slutty shirt. Maybe then. I won't. Be fat. Or maybe I'll be a fat girl in too-tight jeans.

I'm meeting my body image group for dinner at some chain restaurant. I think of that overplayed song in which Alanis Morissette asks, "Isn't it ironic?" and isn't it? A bunch of anorexics and bulimics getting together for dinner, me in my new screaming-sex jeans meeting a group of disordered young girls. I wish I was meeting some rugged man with a husky voice, husky from too many cigarettes and too much booze, and I wish he'd throw me against the wall, hold my arms over my head and fuck me, my hair in my face, shoulders pressed back against the wall, bruising.

I haven't eaten at one of these big chain restaurants since middle school, when I was young enough to think this crappy American run-of-the-mill shit-for-food was good. But who cares, so I go.

Everybody likes my jeans. *You look hot!* they tell me. The girls all order salads but I get pasta with chicken in a cream sauce. Hell yeah! I'm fat anyway, so who cares? One girl almost starts crying because she doesn't know what to order. I spend a minute trying to coddle her, to tell her *Aww sweetie pie, just have some food; it's gonna be okay,* but I quickly grow irritated. I'm sick of this shit, these girls who are crying over their dinners (Just eat!), so I shut the fuck up, sip my Diet Coke, and snack on the bread they put out on the table. Another girl passes around photos of her friends. She's still in college. Wow, college. I never had that kind of college life. I flash back to Saturday nights in Boulder: reggae on the radio, or maybe renting a movie with Christopher and baking garlic bread. Some cookie dough from the grocery store. Comfortable sex and early sleep. But this girl's got photos of blonde southern babes in formal dresses. I never even went to prom.

Actually I did go to prom, once, but it doesn't count. There was no corsage, no champagne, no limo, and no hotel room. Certainly no dinner before with friends. No dinner at all, actually. No dress shopping, no updo or makeup. Well, maybe mascara and lip gloss. It was early in high school, my boyfriend Drew invited me, but his school wasn't a real school; it was an "alternative" school, which meant that nobody went to class anyway, and when they did show up they didn't do any actual work, and you were allowed to smoke cigarettes in the hallways, or maybe not, but it seemed that way. And he only went for a year or two and didn't graduate, and so the prom was like fifteen people, maybe twenty, in a big bright room with some tables and plastic chairs. All the guys wore jeans and some of the girls did, too. We stayed about an hour and then drove around town looking for some other friends.

I'm grateful when dinner at this stupid effing restaurant is over so I can get in my truck and drive home. Charlotte walks with me through the parking lot, and we talk hurriedly about what a ridiculous event *that* was and make plans to meet at Arch's the next night.

I'm depressed when I get home. I'm depressed that I'm home. I'm depressed that I'm fat in tight jeans. I'm depressed that these lame girls can't eat some damn food. I'm depressed that I'm as lame as they are. I'm depressed so I'm eating from my fridge, standing in the kitchen, still wearing my hot jeans, shoveling organic chocolate chips in my mouth in spoonfuls with organic peanut butter, washing it down with organic soy milk, light, and going to bed without brushing my teeth, without masturbating. This is the life.

If this is the life, check me out, please. Check me out soon. If this is the life, crying in your food, friendless, sexless, fat, if this is the life, living down the road from your parents, if this is the life, unemployed, alone, scared. If this is the life. Check me out. Check me out, please, check me out soon.

# JANUARY 18, 2003

I'm standing in my client's home gym, looking out the big windows at the beautiful Virginia countryside. It's 9:00 A.M. on a snowy day in January, and I feel pretty happy. My moods have been up and down lately. It's almost as if I believe in myself for long enough to surge forward, but as soon as I doubt myself for some reason, I'm sent spiraling downward into a deep depression. My mom is still here to soothe me, and Anne reminds me that this is pretty normal: that complete recovery from an eating disorder takes years. I've decided that the only way to really recover is to be authentic to myself, so I'm taking my moods in stride, as best I can.

Personal training, it turns out, is not triggering me. It's helping me. I want to be a good example for my clients. Sometimes they get emotional; sometimes they cry. I'm not the only one who houses pain in her body. One of my clients hasn't worked out since her brother died. When I put her on the stationary bicycle in her makeshift gym, she starts crying within the first few minutes. How do I feel when this happens? I'm proud of her. I'm moved. I can relate. The body, I'm discovering, despite how it participated in my illness, can also be a source of healing. Movement isn't solely about burning calories or building muscle; movement is about healing.

This doesn't mean that I've made a sudden transformation and no longer run or punish myself through workouts. I still do. But I'm conscious now; I'm thinking about it differently. I'm stopping earlier, almost as soon as I stop enjoying it.

My client walks into the room, and I'm pulled from my daydreams out the wintry Virginia window. She's wearing a beautiful exercise outfit, something so flattering and stylish, almost dancerly, that I momentarily feel too sporty and athletic in my ponytail and warm-up pants. Our dialogue is friendly. She's traveled a lot, lived all over the world, and as I train her we talk about her husband, her career shifts, her children. I'm learning that being trainer also means playing therapist. I listen and nod, laugh when appropriate, and try to keep her focused on the exercises. *Watch your back, engage your abs, okay, Susan? Good, one more time.* I feel competent, confident, strong.

## FEBRUARY 16, 2003

I'm flip-flopping a lot these days. Some weeks I am strong, confident, and well. But other weeks I still feel disordered, depressed, and unable to pick myself up. On a confident whim, I decide to fly to Los Angeles to meet Charlotte and her roommate Claire, who are taking a big West Coast trip. It's a last-minute decision, but I have nothing else to do. I don't have the money, but that's what credit cards are for, so I book a ticket and head on out. When I arrive in LA my confidence plummets, and I spend most of the time feeling crummy.

I'm wearing the same tight jeans I bought last month at Wet Seal. I arrive several hours before Charlotte and Claire and take a bus all over the city until it drops me at the home of a friend of Claire's from high school. His name is Carl. He's a skinny LA rocker with an LA rocker haircut and an LA rocker dog: something tiny, in an abusive-looking collar, that yaps and shits and licks. I can't sleep in Carl's house; I'm on some cushions on the floor, with Claire and Charlotte on couches near me, and the whole place smells.

On our second day I decide to get a room at the Standard Hotel in Hollywood, which I'm told is the same hotel, but maybe not the same location, where the *Sex and the City* girls stayed on their LA trip episode. I remember it; they keep a model in a glassed-in cage behind the reception desk, and the character Samantha is impressed. I'm pretty impressed, too, walking in. This is definitely *so LA*. For some reason it's only about $100 a night, maybe $150, and makes my visit so much more enjoyable. I watch TV, take baths, and sit by the pool. I wonder why I'm in LA. I could do this at home, minus the pool since it's the middle of February, but it would be free.

Charlotte and Claire go with Carl and his friends to clubs to see music while I stay in my hotel room, order room service, and binge on candy bars. They go shopping and buy designer jeans, funky shoes, and jewelry. I tag along for the shopping but don't buy anything. I just wish I was home.

I'm constipated the whole short trip and have insomnia. I take a laxative one night and spend the next morning, on almost no sleep, whimpering and alternating between the bathtub and the toilet. Charlotte and I have a couple great moments, just the two of us; after all, that's when we're really at our best. One afternoon we hike high up in the Hollywood Hills and swear Cameron Diaz drives past us in her little hybrid car. We love the exercise, the way our butts feel the next day. Another afternoon we drive around, just us, in Claire's rental car. We're going to pick her up at some art school she's visiting. We cruise around, blasting music, drinking frappuccinos.

But other than those two moments, I wish I was at home. Miserable at home. Miserable with my mom at home. Twenty-three years old. Miserable and homesick in Los Angeles. Feeling fat, for sure; it's like MTV beach party all over the place. My sexy tight jeans definitely make me look fat in this crowd, and I didn't even bring any makeup. What am I doing here?

I fly home, with a bad cold, and spend one night in Charlottesville before flying up to Boston.

# February 26, 2003

Nat and Katy are a disgusting couple. They smoke in the house, and she's unemployed. There's garbage everywhere, pots with hardened rice sitting in the sink, and rotting food left out on the table. Their cat sheds everywhere and I'm allergic, making the situation that much more repugnant.

But still, I'm glad to be visiting. It's cold and snowy in Boston, and I'm wearing my favorite long coat and big cozy sweaters. I sleep on a futon mattress on the living room floor. They stay up late. Exceedingly late. Katy does things like cut and dye Nat's hair at 4:00 A.M., a cigarette hanging from her lip, in her underwear. There's a carton of open doughnuts on the desk, by the ashtray full of cigarette butts. The cat is between their feet. They're laughing hysterically. They're drunk.

I watch. Because I have to. I have nowhere else to go. It's my last night here, thank god; I'm leaving in the morning, assuming the snow doesn't interfere. I came up to Boston to give another poetry reading at WordsWorth Books in Harvard Square, at the invitation of my kind friend Joshua. And, of course, I hoped to see Aaron.

And I did. Someone asks, *Why didn't you invite him to the poetry reading?* Which is a ridiculous question. Aaron and I are lovers first, friends a steep second. So we made plans for earlier tonight. He took me to this restaurant in Allston, some sports bar I've never heard of, and when he dropped me off back at Nat's, he whipped out his cock and said, *Suck it, baby.* I laughed in his face. This was one of many nights of laughing in Aaron's face in the car, him pulling his dick out, asking me to perform some sexual favor like we're in the beginning of a really hot porno flick. But we're not. I don't know where he's been, I don't want any diseases, so I said I wouldn't suck it, but I did touch it. Momentarily. Then he took over, came on his clothes, and kissed me goodnight. I let myself into Nat's place and told him and Katy the story. Then I ate ice cream and climbed into bed.

Now it's 9:00 P.M., and Nat and Katy are appalled. Nat tells me I remind him of our least favorite neighbor from growing up, the depressing one who kept old trunks in her attic, and that I need to let a little life back into my, well, my life. I think he's encouraging me to live like him and Katy, constantly drunk and saying stupid things to bartenders, but somewhere in there he's got a point. If I live out of fear constantly, I'm going to be depressed. Which I am. *But I gave a great poetry reading last night!* Nat doesn't dispute this but argues that life can be good every day, not just once a month or so.

I put on lipstick and a sexier shirt. We catch a cab over to Cambridge and go to the Enormous Room, a bar I've been to once before. When I walk in, the bouncer grabs my ass and gives me his card.

I get drunk on mai tais. In the middle of the winter! I smoke cigarettes, I flirt with men, I eat at 2:00 A.M. on our way home. But the next day I fly back to Virginia, and my life is much of the same.

## MARCH 19, 2003

Mom and I are standing together in the post office at Barracks Road Shopping Center. I've just returned from a session with my morning client, and I'm wearing purple spandex dance pants and a pink zip-up hoodie. I'm explaining to Mom that I want to train for a triathlon, and I promise it's for the right reasons. She's carrying a handful of packages to send Tor at school and is asking me to remind her to buy a roll of stamps. I'm thinking I can't ever imagine needing to buy a whole roll of stamps at one time, and how Mom always kept a roll in the cupboard above her kitchen desk, my entire childhood. Now she keeps them at her studio, in the second drawer on the left. I know this because I steal them whenever I need to mail something. I also steal small change from the studio store, but this is beside the point at the moment because I desperately want my mother's approval on this triathlon issue.

*Talk it over with Anne.* That's what she finally concludes. Everything since my eating disorder's inception seems to be left in Anne's hands, and I wonder if Anne has any idea how much weight she carries in terms of my life choices. It's true that she's my most reliable sounding board—my dietitian turned life coach—and if I get her approval I'll feel like I really do want to be in the race for the right reasons. After all, I'm a trainer now, educating other people on fitness and wellness. My approach with my clients is moderate, joyful, and supportive. I can take that same approach with myself, can't I?

Anne says okay. The day I visit her office—she's in a different office now than when I first met her—it's drizzling outside. She gets excited with me, even, about how much fun I'll have. And she points out that the sprint distance triathlon I want to do isn't that far outside what I'm already comfortable doing. *You could do it today, Peach, so don't train too hard.*

# April 1, 2003

I borrow a bike from a friend. I practice swimming and running on the same day. I practice running farther. I practice swimming farther. I get used to the bike and I get it tuned up and I ride to the gym where I swim and then I run and I ride my bike home and in no time it's strange but my shoulder injury is back and in no time it's strange but my right knee hurts every time I climb stairs and in no time it's strange but my left elbow hurts my elbow has never hurt before and something is wrong with my foot and in no time I'm back in the sports medicine clinic and my doctor is shaking his head and I have tendonitis in several places, in every important joint on at least one side of my body and *You're this close,* he says, *to a stress fracture in your left foot,* and then, *Why were you training so hard for such a short race, Peach? You were already fit enough to do it without all this work!*

Why was I training so hard. For such a short race.

For the excuse, for a reason, for a way to let myself push to exhaustion and push further, for a reason to overeat at lunch and a reason to work out twice or three times in one day, for a way to justify it, to not just be an overexercising freak but to be an athlete, to have a legitimate goal, to tell everyone, *I'm training for a triathlon* instead of *I just like to run,* to prove to the world that all my hard work isn't just about having a certain body and to be able to sleep well at night, to sleep knowing that I have a real goal in life, a purpose, because nothing I'm doing feels like it's getting me anywhere I want to go or anywhere valid or worthy at all. The rest of my life feels full of anxiety and fear and all I can detect is time passing and the numbing of my feet on the sidewalk. *I swear,* I told my mother, I told Anne, *it's not the eating disorder that wants to be in the race.*

# MAY 3, 2003

I'm collapsed on the floor at Mom's studio, in her assistant Bethany's office, crying my eyes out to her my skirt is flailing around my waist I'm throwing a genuine temper tantrum, one of what feels like many in the last few years, I can feel the sweat from my crying all salty down my shirt and on my face I have sworn off exercise, really, truly, a real break, I swear it, I promise, my knees hurt, my hips hurt, my feet hurt, I can't move my shoulder I have beaten my body for years and now I have to stop but still by 3:00 P.M. I'm hysterical it's withdrawal I can't work out today I know I can't I haven't now for three days and I have to take the whole summer off I feel like I'm dying I'm crying in Bethany's lap she comforts me it works I love her I love being in someone's arms and afterward I go to a movie with Jane and it feels better, it does, to rest.

# MAY 2003

I do my best to hide my injuries from my clients. I'm embarrassed. I spend so much time with my clients talking about injury prevention, about the necessity of rest, about cross-training and listening to your body. I do finally confess to one older client that I've got some knee pain from running, because I can't demonstrate a squat for her right now, but other than that, I think I manage to keep my pain silent during training sessions.

It's no fun—beautiful Virginia spring and I have to rest! The air is amazingly thick right now: sweet smelling, with buds opened and petals fluttering around car tires driving through town. I hang out with Mom at the studio, help her with the phones and other administrative details when I'm not with my clients. I actually have only a few clients: three, sometimes four (one woman lives half-time in Charlottesville and half-time in New York). So there's plenty of time outside of that to work at Studio 206 and help my mom. But I'm still fairly selfish with my time, and I still keep my cottage immaculately clean.

# June 17, 2003

I love riding a bike in a skirt. Today I'm wearing a stretchy blue one, navy with lighter blue flowers, the flowers taking up most of the skirt, with a white T-shirt and pink flip-flops. Mom and I have been taking morning rides up and down the island. I'm not counting this as exercise since it's really just leisure, the equivalent of a stroll. We go slowly and stop to read historic signs. One day we walk into the lighthouse shop and another morning we try to find the house we stayed in our first summer here, but neither of us can remember it well enough. We do find the right street, but it's all fuzzy to me. I was fifteen or sixteen that summer and brought my boyfriend Drew with us. He took nude photographs of me in the tide pools at low tide. A few years later they showed up on the walls of an art gallery and I called the owner to have them taken down. Almost regretfully—they were beautiful photographs, black and white, my soft curvy teenage body melding with the water.

The tide pools are one of my favorite parts of Bald Head Island. When the big ocean mouth recedes, all these giant puddles form on the beach, some big enough to swim across, all of them warm and soft and silky. Islands form out in the ocean, too; our favorite is Pelican Island, and people swim out to it during low tide. I never have, but Dad and I talk about it all the time. It's not a particularly challenging swim, but it's far enough out that it makes us both a little nervous. I love the way water feels, and I'm a strong swimmer, but the ocean scares me a bit. My mom's father drowned in the ocean when she was only two, and I'm sure her own fears about the sea informed the way she raised my brother and me when we were kids on the beach. While all my friends ran and dove into the ocean, I held back a bit. I'm in my twenties now and I don't have a problem swimming in the ocean anymore, especially on the water here near Cape Fear, off the coast of North Carolina, because it's so warm. But I want a more courageous partner than my father. We decide to go for it one moment, and the next he asks, *What about the sharks?* There are sharks here, but I don't think they'll bite us. They aren't that big.

We spend most of our Bald Head mornings on the beach and most of the afternoons napping. It's always oppressively hot here, and we laugh at ourselves for how much we love it despite the heat. At night, after dinner, we drive the golf cart around sipping gin and tonics, or else pile everyone in (Victoria always brings a friend) and putt on over to near where the ferry docks to get ice cream cones. These are some of my favorite Bald Head moments: licking an ice cream cone in the rocking chairs outside the sweet shop, Tor and her friend of choice finding some teenage boys to flirt with, watching the sun set.

This summer, Mom and I have incorporated bike rides into the daily schedule despite my knee pain, which is keeping me from most other activities. In fact, I have to hobble, jumping a little, keeping most of the weight on my left leg, to get up the stairs to my loft apartment over the golf-cart garage. But the bike doesn't bother it, and I like the time alone with Mom. Being with Mom is almost always leisurely; time slows down, and we don't rush. I'm in a good mood when we pull back up to our beach house. Dad's sitting on the porch, and I grab a piece of fruit before I realize he has a sort of dumbfounded expression on his face. Like he's been defeated.

*The girls took the golf cart—they went off with those older boys.* My heart is pounding. Tor and her friend have been hanging out with eighteen-year-olds, and they're only fourteen, about to be high school freshmen, and I know the difference between a fourteen-year-old and an eighteen-year-old. The difference is sex. Eighteen-year-old boys have sex, want sex, see girls as a means to an end. Fourteen-year-old girls want sex, too, but they don't always know what it involves. Their twenty-three-year-old sisters do, though, and my heart starts to race with the force of true adrenalin. I'm flashing back to being fifteen and sixteen years old on the beach with a high school friend, vacationing somewhere on the Outer Banks with her family. I'm remembering sneaking out, drinking beer with men in their thirties, and the way one kept grabbing my tits, kissing my mouth. I'm remembering running away from them, drunk, and thinking later that it was a genuine close call. A close call that not everyone escaped: I'm mentally listing all my girlfriends who were raped or assaulted in high school. I hate that it's an actual list, but it is.

The fact is, Tor doesn't keep secrets from me. She snuck out last night, with her friend, and met these same boys at the grocery store. Mom and Dad are oblivious. Dad thinks Tor can do no wrong; she's his princess. *She's a teenager,* I tell him, but he doesn't take it in. I guess I understand that. What parent wants to face the facts? But this older sister does. It's all I can face.

I ask Dad if he got their address, and he did. I'm pissed she has the golf cart, I'm pissed nobody else realizes how serious this is, and I tear off on the bike back down the island, this time on the beach side rather than through the trees, where Mom and I rode just a little while ago. I make it about halfway when the chain comes off the spokes, and I get my hands all greasy in the sand trying to put it back on. Two men stop to help, my urgency attracting their attention. I finally reach the older boys' street, pass over a little bridge, and check momentarily for crocodiles. Then I throw the bike in the sand, bound up the stairs (knee pain, what knee pain?), and burst into the house without knocking.

There sit my sister and her friend, on a couch opposite the couch where the three older boys sit. The TV is on. My fire should be quenched: Clearly I overreacted. But it isn't. Seeing these boys with their shirts off in the same room with my sister just makes my blood boil even faster. I tell them I came to get the golf cart. I tell them I'm leaving the bike, oh, and by the way, the chain is falling off. I'm warming up for my speech. My mouth is dry. *Do you know how old these girls are?* I ask the boys. I know they don't; I know Tor said they were sixteen. They nod. *Look,* I say, hands on my hips, sweaty hair in my face, *I may not look tough, but I am*—the boys are looking at me, standing in the doorway of their beach house—*and I'll cut your fucking balls off if you touch them.*

Tor's mouth falls open and she guffaws, seriously. She looks half thrilled by me, sort of proud almost, and also horrified. I walk out of the house, leaving the broken bike, and drive the golf cart back to my parents' cottage, where they wait with eyes open wide, wondering what absurd thing Peach might have done now. The ride back is sort of a downer; I miss the forcefulness of physical exertion. Our golf cart putters pretty slowly, as is the point, and I'm plugging it back into the wall to charge when Dad says, *So? How'd it go?*

Tor and I talk about it that night. I confide, *Tor, boys will hurt you, boys hurt me.* I tell her things I haven't told her before, but I can't remember exactly what. Maybe how my first boyfriend would have sex with me while I was passed out drunk in the guest bedroom of someone's house whose parents were out of town. Maybe I tell her about my childhood friend being raped. Maybe I tell her how amazing sex finally was with Christopher, when we knew how to take care of each other. Whatever I tell her, I know my point is clear: We make choices when we're young without understanding the consequences. I have been through almost a decade of therapy at this point, I have had an eating disorder, and all of this is based in pain, partly pain from choices I made when I was her age.

She giggles—she is both mad and thrilled by what I did and said to those boys. I apologize. I overreacted. But my concern doesn't fade. I realize yet again how scary it is to love someone. I love my sister with so much force, more than I've ever loved anyone, and I want to help her, to mold her, to make sure she doesn't make the choices that I made, that my friends made. But I also realize that she isn't me; she has her own body and her own mind, and she has to learn for herself. This breaks my heart, and I spend the next morning lying in the sand, crying to Mom about Christopher. *I can't believe I'm still crying about Christopher,* I tell her. But she enforces that I'm not crying about Christopher, I'm crying about myself.

I spend the rest of the week baking peach cobblers and cheesecakes. In my summer off of exercise, I'm really embracing food. I try out things Mom never let me have as a kid: white bread with the kind of peanut butter that doesn't separate. I put cream and sugar in my coffee and eat Oreos in bed at night. I've gained weight, I'm my heaviest ever, but it doesn't bother me. I'm relaxed most of the time and enjoying being with my family.

The boys show up at our house the last night of vacation, and Mom makes me offer them a piece of cake. I do, but then I say, *Remember the other day? I meant what I said.* I have to have the last word, but it feels weakened now; all the strength of that moment in their house has faded into another piece of my depression, a pathetic desperation. And that seems clear to everyone, even these teenage boys sitting on our back porch with the ceiling fan turning. My sister's big smile, her braces gleaming. I retreat back into the house to cut myself a big slice of cake and then sit with Mom and Dad on the front porch, sipping gin and tonics.

# JULY 8, 2003

I haven't had sex in a year but I want to tonight, desperately—I can feel it early on. I go with Mom to a movie, but it's so hot—it's July in Virginia, it's the weather for sex. I don't have many friends; I have a few, but I don't know where they are, so I don't call them. After the movie I drive to Whole Foods to buy sushi.

I'm heavier than I've been in a while. Ever? I'm softer, too. My body is curvy; Jane says I look like a goddess. I'm slowly getting used to my shape, my size. Slowly learning to accept my appetite for its lustiness and my body for her roundness, her plumper parts.

Tonight has the softest air. I'm wearing a skirt that brushes my legs and I love the way it feels—a pretty, peasanty, hippie skirt in browns and reds, with a red tube top my sister gave me for my birthday last year. I haven't exercised this summer, and the relaxation is bringing sex back into my body. Everything is making my skin stand on end tonight: the air-conditioning in the movie theater, the way the canvas of my truck seat scratches at the backs of my arms, the vibrating sensation in the gearshift, and the tickle my hair makes across my forehead.

When I pull into the lot, I park facing another pickup and watch a sexy, rugged Virginia man step out. Smoke. All through my body. Suddenly. Who is he? He sees me. Immediately. There must be smoke all around my body. He's a little shorter than I usually go for. But I'm pretty sure I can get over it. Look at his arms. Look at his old T-shirt. Why is that so hot? I bet his hands are calloused. I want them to cut my body.

I climb out of my truck I do it silently screaming sex and I swear the whole shopping center must be able to smell my desire

I am unable to contain it and I walk the way a woman in heat walks, she can't help it, I can't help it, I move toward that door and I eye him and he sees me the whole time and when I step in front of the sliding glass entranceway I have to stop. Whole Foods is closed. He stops, too; he's at the opposite entrance, facing me. We turn. We walk. Back to our trucks. We both drive trucks. I'm imagining what he smells like I can tell already, his hair is thick and blonde his chest is thick his arms are thick he could hold me down hard he could do whatever he wanted I climb into my truck I look at him he raises his arm toward me—

*Where can I get a bottle of wine around here?* I look at his truck. Hawaii license plates! I give him directions. We start our engines. I think, *What, that's it? I know you want more I can smell it on your rugged skin I can smell the dirt and sweat from here I know you want more.* We pull our trucks out and they're side by side at the stoplight. He's turning left. I'm turning right. My window is down, my fingers are in my hair, and I'm about to pull away. *This is your last fucking chance if you want the best lay of your life* I'm thinking *God damn I am the easiest woman in Charlottesville tonight all you have to do is—*

*Do you want to get a drink?* He's talking to me. Out the window of his truck, into the window of mine. I turn. I pause. I swear I'm the hottest woman alive. *What's your name?* I ask. *Pull over,* he insists. *Follow me,* I respond.

We pull into a bank parking lot. His name is Kurt. My name is Peach; he doesn't smile or think it's interesting. He wants me to come to his house and a little of my fever is put out: I'm horny, okay, but buy me a drink first, I need a little courting. I tell him I don't even know him. *I know this bar,* he tells me. I know it—it's a total dive, nobody goes there, it's right by the miniature golf course where Christopher and I would play with our high school friends. The bar will be empty, and that's fine. I follow him there.

Isn't Charlottesville great? I know his mother. My parents are friends with his mother. We figure this out about twenty minutes into our drink, and I learn that he's thirty, that he just moved back after spending three years in Hawaii. He works construction; he knows another kid I know, who works with him. That and the fact that his mother is a perfect, blonde, country club woman is how I justify going home with him after we finish our rum and Cokes. He is nothing like his mother. He turns on a movie but his face is under my skirt so fast and he takes breaks only to drink more beer from the twelve-pack he stopped for on the way to his apartment and suddenly I'm doubting myself and pushing away but then I ask, *Peach, what did you come here for, if not this very moment?*

His bed is amazing. Why do all men, even the ones who don't shower enough or shave enough or clean their rooms have amazingly soft sheets, amazing pillows, incredibly perfect mattresses? Creature comfort. Men. Creature comfort.

We fuck. It's heavenly. He holds me down like I knew he would, he forgets my name, he calls me Rose, I don't care, he has a tattoo on his ankle and a surfboard in the corner of his room. We fuck all night and into the morning he fucks me so slowly but with so much control and power it's the best sex I've ever had, I know it, which is maybe only because it's been a year and I wanted it so bad but also because he's got the perfect marriage of skills: absolute authority and absolute tenderness. I come maybe three times, I can't remember. I'm woken up by him inside me; I don't sleep at all. We use a condom the first time and after that it's forgotten. I quiz him on his health: *When is the last time you were tested blah blah who is your doctor*—and of course, don't you love Charlottesville, I know his fucking doctor. In the morning he grabs me by the ankles and pulls me to the edge of the bed and fucks me again and at some point I give him my phone number and then I drive away straight to a cafe for a huge muffin and a coffee and look around and watch everyone heading to work in straight pants and I think, *I just had the best sex of my life, you motherfuckers, and you don't even know.*

I go home and call my mother to tell her, sitting on the front walk of my cottage, fingering the flowers and grass, knowing I need to mow the lawn. *Hey, Mom, I had sex last night with your friend's son.*

<center>~~~</center>

He never called. I got a cold and then an HIV test a few months later, which was negative, thank god. I remembered later that he stopped at some point during the night to tell me how much he loved my body, its voluptuousness, my curves, and I realized that's all I needed from him. Charlotte and I drove by his house one night and his truck was there, and then we went for frozen yogurt. He never called. But I was on again, lit and ready for more. Screw exercise, screw diets; men love my luscious body and I love them in it. Welcome to heartache, welcome to real life again, welcome to sex with orgasms and endless nights of waiting for the phone to ring. But good-bye isolation, good-bye illness, good-bye craving control over freedom. Welcome back, Peach.

# AUGUST 9, 2003

I meet Peter at a party for Charlottesville's yearly "Best of" competition. Studio 206 is once again winning Best Yoga Studio, but I think this year they're calling it "Best Place to Align Your Chakras." I've just started working this shitty temp job at some financial place and meet up with Mom, Dad, and Bethany for the party at South Street. South Street is a popular bar, mellow, very Virginia. When I was a kid it was more of a restaurant, or maybe that's the kid's perspective. We used to go there in the fall for crabs. Yum.

I'm feeling pretty hot, still all sexified from my one-night stand with Kurt the Whole Foods guy and from hours of rubbing my thigh-highed and gartered legs together under my desk in a fatally boring desk job. I'm wearing a black and white polka-dot skirt, a little too tight now since I bought it years ago at a completely different weight. With a black tank top, also tight, and black heels, hair all curly and in my face. I'm snacking at the buffet, palming a beer, and chatting with my parents' friends. This really, really tall guy is eying me. Tall is good. The bigger the better: The bigger the man, the smaller I feel. Now there's a nod or something—not a smile, we don't smile, but we sort of half nod, and he walks over to me and introduces himself. *Hey, I'm Peter,* he says. *Who are you here with?* I tell him I'm Chris Friedman's daughter and here with Studio 206 to accept the little award thing. The plaque. Whatever they give you. He tells me he's a writer and asks if he can catch up with me later; for now he wants to mingle and schmooze. I smile and go find Bethany, bosom up to her and order another beer. Point him out from across the room. *He's tall!* Bethany says.

Mom and Dad leave after the awards, but I stay for a while, and Peter and I finally grab a table together by the bar. I'm thinking, *Good, he'll take me back to his place and we'll make out all night.* Instead, he asks me for my number. Why don't men know how easy I am?

He calls the next afternoon, while I'm at Anne's for an appointment, actually. We decide to see a movie later, and he puts his arm around me in the theater and kisses me goodnight beside my truck, back in the parking lot behind Studio 206. I want more. I want everything. All the time. But he is shy.

# AUGUST 11, 2003

I recently got a new job. I had to. The thought had entered my head again—it happens every couple of months. Mom hates whenever I get like this; she doesn't want me to take crap work to make money. She is so not all about settling, and I love her for it, because it means she'll give me money unless I'm doing work I love. I am training a few clients, still, and I do love that work, but I feel so inadequate compared to my friends with real jobs in cities like San Francisco and Boston. (I did that, didn't I, but it feels like a lifetime ago!) Besides that, I'm broke.

So I convince myself, and maybe it is time. I've had a summer laying off exercise, I've played around with friends, eaten ice cream constantly, helped Mom out at work and trained a few clients a week, but I'm getting a little stir crazy for *direction* and *success* and wouldn't mind some cash. Seriously. Like, now. So about a week before that Best Of party I went back to my old reliable friend, the friend that got me through my semester off in college and the low points in Boulder when I wasn't living within my allowance: the temp agency. They love me because I can type like a fiend; in fact, on this go-round the agent asks me to take the typing test *again* because she doesn't trust that the 112 words per minute I score is accurate. The second time I get 115. I've also lived in Boston now, don't forget, and worked as an executive administrative assistant (it sounds so . . . totally not glamorous, so miserable), so I'm experienced for mundane office work, and they give me a job at some company that certifies financial professionals, I think. I never fully get what the company does, but I buy a suit at Ann Taylor for the interview, and that's the fun part. I also buy thigh-highs with garters and a pair of heels. If I'm going to work in an office again, I'm going to at least look the part—that is, the part played by the girl who fantasizes constantly about giving blow jobs under desks and flirts with the men who deliver the mail or work in shipping and receiving.

I thought that secretarial job at UVa's hospital was the worst ever, but this one takes the cake. It's worse because I'm a temp, so I have no salary, no benefits, no ID badge. My cube is out in the open, and I have no idea what I do, except type in a bunch of crap they want me to type, and again, I do it so fast they run out of work to give me, so I mostly e-mail Charlotte. Luckily, her boss is out of town, so she e-mails back. I've just started dating Peter, and I e-mail him, too, and then I forward all the e-mails he writes me back on to Charlotte to analyze them. She does, and I'm left cracking up at my desk, thigh-highs and garters shifting under my skirt, waiting for my lunch break. Or the end of the day, please, the end of the day.

While Charlotte's boss is out of town she meets me for long lunches that often end with a stop at Arch's. I leave the office for two hours at a time and could care less. We're getting Arch's twice a day now: once at lunch and once after dinner. We read the local newspapers and magazines while we're sitting there, spooning frozen yogurt and gooey brownies into our mouths. When I get back to work I feel like I'm going to die.

I start exercising again. It's the only way to get by. Simple stuff: a two-mile jog here and there, sometimes during lunch when Charlotte can't get away (she never can when her boss is around) and sometimes after work, before I meet up with Charlotte for dinner and Arch's. If I don't feel like jogging, I go to Andrew's yoga class at Mom's studio. I have a huge crush on him. He's hot. He's a poet, too, a rare combination. I love his legs, his arms; I love when he comes around and puts his hands on my body to adjust my pose or help me relax. Once or twice Charlotte comes with me to yoga, but usually I go alone and then meet her afterward. For dinner. And Arch's.

## AUGUST 29, 2003

I start thinking I'll invite Peter, who I'm now calling my dating partner because he's not my boyfriend, to a yoga class, but I never do. My dating partner and I don't really see each other all that often, or talk all that often, but we have some fun. At least he's someone to hang out with if Charlotte has other plans. The sex is mediocre: He's not aggressive enough. The first time we really made out I had to force him into the bedroom, and then he went soft on me and that was pretty much that. He spends the night sometimes, but I don't love the way he smells, which should have been a clear indicator right away. Usually I fall in love with men by the third date because I'm already addicted to their smell. This never happens with Peter, but we keep dating because he's the only man in my age group in Charlottesville who I didn't go to high school with, or who one of my friends hasn't fucked. In fact, I don't know of anyone who Peter's fucked, and maybe that should have been a warning sign, but Charlotte says she had a friend from college who did an internship with him a few years ago and had a crush on him.

I last at the temp job only a few weeks. I leave in a very disrespectful manner, as I'm getting comfortable doing, at least since the UVa job. I just walk out. One day at lunch, even! I'm looking around the office and at this piece of paper in my hand, which I'm supposed to do something with, but I don't know what, and I leave. I go home, go for a run, and never go back. I briefly consider returning because I left some snacks in my desk drawers, but I can steal more money from Mom, or from the studio, and replace those Luna bars and the jar of peanut butter.

I do at least e-mail and say I won't be returning. The lady at the temp agency is pretty disappointed in me; she scolds me and insists that I not do that again, but I'm a hot commodity in the Charlottesville temp pool, what with that typing score and all, so she lines me up pretty fast in a much better position: as a legal assistant for a small firm downtown.

# SEPTEMBER 8, 2003

Kids are going back to school. I have my own office at the firm, which kind of makes me feel like I'm back in Boston. My boss here appreciates me. He gives me work; he commends what I do with it. I learn quickly, and I enjoy the office dynamics. Every day at lunch I meet my high school friend Lindsay, who is interning at a design firm a couple of blocks away, in the park between our two offices. And every morning before work, I run.

I'm back in shape. It took about a month, but I can do my six-mile loop again, and it feels good. I'm also on a diet. An extreme one. I started it about a week ago, and I've cut out several food groups: meat, most notably. The only dairy I'll eat is yogurt and cottage cheese. No butter, no matter what. No cheese, no matter what. And all oils and fats extremely sparingly. No processed foods. A lot of tea. A lot of miso soup, even though it's still hot out. A lot of this new wrap I sort of invented: a sprouted wheat tortilla with hummus, a sheet of nori, sliced cabbage, sliced carrot, sliced tomato, sprouts, and a tiny, tiny drizzle of olive oil. I eat this at lunch with Lindsay, with an apple. I'm losing weight.

I defend my diet to my mother as a means to cure my chronic constipation, which I have suffered from since the second half of my year in Boston. I cannot, for the life of me, take a shit under pressure. Which means that whenever I take these temp jobs, I will go weeks without eliminating anything I've eaten. It can't be healthy, and it's painful. When I'm unemployed, or employed at Studio 206 making my own hours, I don't feel rushed or anxious and my body relaxes and I shit. This is a disgusting and embarrassing problem, but it keeps me from employment, has kept me from employment, and I can't deal any longer. Hence the major dietary changes, and it works. Because despite having a job where I do have to appear in the office by 9:00 A.M. and be there until 5:00 P.M., generally, I'm eating mostly vegetables and fruits, so things just *move*. I discuss this with Lindsay endlessly. My life is so mundane.

# SEPTEMBER 21, 2003

I'm losing weight and it's autumn. The mornings are cooler, so I enjoy my runs even more. Then I make oat bran for breakfast and chamomile tea in a big mason jar that I carry to work. Charlotte is a little fed up with me, with what I'm doing with food. She notices I've lost weight, but I manage to convince her that it's for the right reasons (she has listened to me complain about my nonfunctioning bowels for long enough). She's supportive, but I can tell it sort of bothers her. As it should.

Peter my dating partner doesn't notice that I lose weight. We go to movies, sometimes dinner. We run into each other at the bars with our friends on Friday nights. We sometimes go a week or two without talking.

## THANKSGIVING 2003

It still feels like every date with Peter is a second date. We have sex but it's nothing to write home about, or even write about at all. Still, I invite him to my parents' Thanksgiving party. Nat comes home for Thanksgiving this year, looking so debonair I can't stand it, in a good way. I love my brother! I am always so proud to be on his arm, so proud to show him off to my friends. He looks fantastic in blue and is wearing a shirt that color and nice dark jeans; he's so citified and I love seeing him. We take a walk together before the party. He's still smoking cigarettes so I smoke one with him, and we gab about Mom and Dad and how they're doing and if we think Tor is hanging in there.

I've lost about twenty pounds and am actually gaining again, or am about to. I think this weight loss is part of a balancing act. It's true that I'm doing my diet to cure constipation, but I'm also experimenting with my hunger and satiety, and not in a terribly risky way. My weight now is back to about where it was before my eating disorder. I don't want to be sick. I don't want to be controlling with food. I want to be happy and well, so I hire a new dietitian, just for a change. I want to work with someone who won't tell me that it's okay to binge, like Anne still tells me. I want one that will help me stay thin. Anne won't do that, and she shouldn't. Her job, she reminds me, why I hired her, she reminds me, was to, is to, cure me, to help me recover from an underweight, anorexic, exercise-obsessed condition. Not to help me stay thin and on some weird vegetarian, fat-free diet. But my new dietitian is okay with me being thin and food picky. I like that. And hate it.

Tor and I go to get our makeup done for the party. She's in braces and has these cute little boobs. We sit on stools at the makeup counter, giggling, drinking our frothy Starbucks concoctions, and talking about boys. How fun to talk with Tor about boys. She has a crush; they talk at night on the phone. She's fourteen years old and lovely.

My daddy throws fabulous parties. He does. The house looks amazing, everyone shows up festive and happy to be there, and Daddy keeps everyone's glass full. Nat has been to India recently on business, in Bangalore, and brought me back this deep blue sari with gold embroidery. At the end of the night, Dad opens the old bottle of Poire William that's sat on the chest in the dining room for years, and we all sip it (*Slowly!* he instructs us). Then Lindsay helps me tie the sari on, and I dance around the big kitchen and fall in Tor's lap on the floor, laughing.

Our kitchen floor holds many memories: That's where I'd sit in the tenth grade when my parents yelled at me for getting bad grades. That's where I'd spread my homework out when I was in elementary school. That's where Mom and I and Nat and Tor and Dad would all sprawl out in the evenings after dinner, laughing and telling jokes and lounging with our golden retriever, Widdie. We are floor people. I'm more comfortable cross-legged on hardwood than I am sitting upright in a chair.

Tonight, relaxing on the floor, now in a sitting position, sipping tea with my back leaning on the cupboards behind me, my family and friends all around, I feel pretty damn good. My heels are sticking out the end of the sari, my hair is messy, and my sister is telling some crude joke and making my friend Jane spit her tea.

*My body,* I think. *Why have I been worrying about my body?* Right now my family seems perfect. We are all here. We are all laughing. We are tipsy on wine and the poire, of course, but also on togetherness, on holidays, on the hardwood floors in our big kitchen. The air outside is pulsing with holiday stars. It's a cold night. I walk outside with Nat while he smokes his last cigarette, and my heart feels full, feels real.

# DECEMBER 11, 2003

It's a cold winter so far. After many months of living back in Virginia, helping Mom out at the studio, dating, training clients, eating frozen yogurt with Charlotte, and continuing to recover, I've decided I'm ready for academia again, for a new challenge. I've decided to apply to graduate programs to earn my MFA in creative writing.

I'm finishing up my applications and have been communicating with a poet at an art school in San Francisco. The idea of moving to the West Coast has never crossed my mind. My ultimate goal is Brown, but its program is tiny and so competitive. My second choice is good ol' UVa. Do I really want to go to school right down the street? I do, but my work is so unconventional, I doubt the Virginia poets really want to claim me as their own. So my old friend Joshua, who hooked me up with those readings in Boston, has put me in touch with an impressive poet in San Francisco who seems to want me at his school. Someone. Wants me? We have e-mailed a bit and set up a late-night phone date to discuss the program (he tells me that this is the great problem of living on the West Coast: His 8:00 P.M. is my 11:00 P.M.). But I do not feel bothered to stay up a little late for this conversation.

*You're already a real poet with a real career,* he tells me on the phone. I'm giddy. *You're exactly the kind of writer we want here.* I have worked so hard for this; if there's anything I've done consistently for my entire literate life, it's write. I'm proud of my work; I believe in poetry, and now someone else believes in me, too. I had plenty of praise at Naropa—it's not like this is the first poet to tell me I'm half decent—but at this point in my life, when I'm so close to a full recovery and so ready for a new adventure, I'm lapping up his words and carrying them with me through my days.

Mom helps me finish my applications. I apply to nine programs altogether, with paperwork spread all over the office floor at Studio 206. I gather my recommendations and put my manuscript together. I sit down with older friends who have MFAs to listen to their advice, their warnings, their successes and struggles. I still hope I'll get into Brown or the University of Virginia, but I feel happy knowing that if those don't work out, California is shaping up to be a worthy option.

# JANUARY 2, 2004

It's a fresh new year, and Peter my dating partner and I are heading to a concert. Really I'm going because I know Christopher will be there. He's back in town visiting his family, and our mutual friends Jane and Lindsay have the word on the street. So I bring Peter because I think it will help me to have a date, even if it's a date I'm not all that into.

Christopher and I hug. I've straightened my long hair and am bundled up but looking cute in a new winter coat and boots. I'm wearing mascara and drinking a beer. He has that same smile on his face: that enormous, genuine, goofy-as-hell smile that makes me weak in the knees, truly. Standing there next to him, catching up, it feels like the same old Christopher and Peach of years past. He is happy to see me, that's clear. He tells me I look great, he makes fun of Peter, and he keeps that damn smile on his face the entire time we talk. It's as if. Nothing has changed? Except that Christopher is in love with another woman. They've been together for a couple of years now, have traveled the world, and it's not as if there's any room for me in his life anymore. Which is okay—at least I think it's okay, until I leave the concert with Peter and he wants me to come back to his house with him, and I really do not want to. It's snowing. I want to go home.

He drops me off, and I eat cookies standing up and then start crying hysterically. I want to call my mother but it's 1:00 A.M. I eventually fall asleep, angry, vulnerable, my long hair wiping the tears from my cheeks and my body quivering under my sheets.

When I wake up I call my mom. She takes me tenderly downtown for a mocha at the Mudhouse, and as we walk around the corner from the studio parking lot, across a small section of the downtown mall, and into our favorite coffee shop, I take a few deep breaths and tell her I still love Christopher.

*Darling, you will always love Christopher,* she tells me, *and he will always love you. But this does not mean that you should be with him. This does not mean that you made a mistake when you left him. This does not mean that anything is out of place in the world. This means only that you are a deep young woman who feels things strongly, who loved a wonderful young man who you happened to see again last night.*

I think. I sip my mocha. I tuck my hair behind my ears. She is right.

*Mommy? I don't want to be with Christopher. That was a long time ago. We were young. I left him because I didn't want our love to go bad. I wanted to always love him. And I still do; I love him as a person and as a man and as someone separate from me. I wish him the best, all the happiness in the world. But I don't want to be with him anymore. I want to find somebody else, somebody who is right for me now, somebody to love as an adult woman, not a young girl.* She pets me, my mom, and we split a big cookie and walk back out into the cold together, climb into her BMW station wagon, and drive over those gentle hills back home to the big house where Daddy has a fire in the fireplace and Tor is upstairs, chatting on the phone with her friends.

# FEBRUARY 4, 2004

Peter my dating partner finally breaks up with me. It's the first time I've ever been broken up with, and I laugh when he tells me.

He stops by my cottage one night because *We need to talk,* he says, and I'm hoping it's a good-bye and thankfully it is—he tells me he met someone special and I laugh and say, *Is it okay that I'm relieved?* And I am. Despite the strong and inevitable human desire to love and be loved, I have greater desires now: to get into graduate school, to stay strong in my recovery, to build a full life that is based in my own dreams and desires.

My eating disorder symptoms are few and far between. I'm not perfect, but I don't worry so much anymore. My body is balancing out. I work out, and I enjoy it. And when I don't want to work out, I don't. I eat normally, and miraculously I shit normally, too. I check in with Anne still, but less often. I have maintained a few clients through my random temp jobs and through my dating escapades, and I enjoy personal training in large part because I love being my own boss. I'm writing and being social in more normal ways. Jane, Lindsay, and I have started a girls craft night, where we alternate houses to make cards or soap or knit, and to eat dinner and cookies, sip tea, gab. I love these women: my strong high school friends who believe in me for me. One afternoon, Charlotte and I throw a winter tea party in my cottage for some local girls. We buy cute petit fours and make a few pots of tea. All the girls arrive in their wellies and sweaters, tromping through the melting snow and up my front walk. I don't freak out because of the mess we make. I am happy to have them in my house, all these sweet Virginia girls and me: a sweet Virginia girl myself, adjusting to being a woman.

# APRIL 5, 2004

Brown, nope. UVa, nope (*I'm sorry, you did not make the short list*). George Mason in Washington, D.C., yes. The New School in NYC—yes, with a scholarship. California College of the Arts in San Francisco—yes, with a huge scholarship. There are others, but none matter now. I'm moving to San Francisco.

Mom is heartbroken. Dad seems pissed. My parents want me close by, and I understand this. They love me. But I have a badass new poet professor in San Francisco who is calling me on the phone and asking me to come to his school, for practically nothing. And an opportunity to live in San Francisco! An adventure.

I think about it. I think about it a lot. New York would be amazing, too, but they aren't offering as much money, and frankly that's a factor now. My parents are sick of supporting me, and I'm sick of taking their money. I don't know anyone in San Francisco. I have only been there once before, with Christopher, on that drive we took back in the summer of 2000 when we took Highway 1 all the way down the coast. All I remember about San Francisco is the smell of urine in the streets and the big public library. Okay, and the homeless people and the sex shops, and honestly the city horrified me. But where better to study poetry than in the lap of the liberal West?

# JUNE 30, 2004

I head to Boston for one last New England hurrah before moving to California. Aaron and I have stayed in touch. Lately, we flirt. He's single, I'm single, it's fun. But our friendship is over the phone; I only see him when I travel to Boston, and it's been a while. I'm excited for this trip because Aaron and I truly love each other now, *as friends*. That doesn't mean I'm not interested in him romantically—I am; our attraction is strong. But it also means we've built the foundation of a real friendship, and I care about him as a person, beyond our flirtation and our sex.

Nat picks me up at the airport. I'm wearing cute jeans and cute sneakers, my hair is straight and blonde, and I look adorable. I'm happy lately. Life is good; there's so much to offer. My family has come around to support my decision to move to California, and my friends are so proud of me. I've come a long way in the last few years, and it feels great to be where I am now: healthy, balanced, and embarking on a new adventure.

Nat has moved into a new apartment on Commonwealth Avenue, a fifth-floor walk-up in the Back Bay. He lives alone now, but his business partner Mason lives in an almost identical apartment on the floor below. Nat and I have a great week together, shopping at Whole Foods, throwing a summer dinner party on the balcony, drinking wine, and laughing. When he's at work, I walk to the Copley mall to shop. I buy a slice of cake in the afternoon, press the back of my fork into the moist, chocolaty dessert, and sigh with happiness. I. Love. Boston. The weather is beautiful, not too hot this week, and we sit outside in the evenings enjoying the air. Nat couldn't be more thrilled about my decision to move to San Francisco: He travels there often for work and loves the city. He has long since broken up with that terrible Katy girl and is single, but really focusing on work. I don't think he's even dating.

I'm not either, really, except that I spend two memorable nights with Aaron this week. The first is just fun: We order frozen yogurt for delivery and talk about personal training. He shows me *a better way to do push-ups* and we have romping sex in his big bed. The second time I see him, he picks me up at Nat's in his truck and takes me to a tapas bar on Beacon Street. We hold hands across the table. He tells me he loves me. I wear this beautiful skirt and gemstone earrings. I nearly tear up at the table. Later, in his bed, he holds me. Aaron has never, ever held me before. He's holding me in his bed. Tenderly. With love, with care. There is no fucking. There is no *suck my cock, baby.* There is only this: *I love you, Peach. You are doing the right thing. You'll be great in San Francisco. You'll never lose me.* I'm crying in his arms, and I can hardly believe the tenderness of our interaction. We have never been this sincere before. He has stood by me as my friend through the ups and downs of my eating disorder, my depression, my exercise addiction and my injuries. He has listened to me whine on the phone about my weight and my fears and my knee pain and my boyfriends, and he has never judged me or stopped caring. But—this is the first time, and it's notable, that he has been so intimate and so tender with me. It's a beautiful, beautiful good-bye.

When I leave his apartment in the morning, it's raining. Nat has booked me two spa appointments at a salon on Newbury Street, and I walk, crying, through the rain. I cry through my facial. I cry through my pedicure. And afterward, I run as fast as I can through the rainy Boston afternoon back to Nat's apartment, up all five flights of stairs, and I sit with a coffee on his balcony, staring at the Prudential Tower, waiting for him to come home. When he does he takes one look at me and says, *You're doing the right thing, Peachie. I love you.*

# JULY 19, 2004

In the realm of eating disorders, relapse is almost guaranteed, and I've slid back a few good yards for every mile I've leaped forward. But right now, getting ready to move to San Francisco, I feel damn near as healthy as I've ever been.

My daddy didn't want me to go so far away at first, but he has come around now and is awfully proud to be sending me off to San Francisco to be a poet. I overhear him tell his friends about it, and it sounds like he's bragging. He even buys me a new car, a little black Jetta with leather seats, to take with me to California. *You need a good city car,* he tells me, but we keep the old pickup in the driveway. Neither of us is quite ready to get rid of it for good.

My dad and I have had a tumultuous relationship. We've argued for most of my life. But the truth is, we're a lot alike. We are both creative and wacky, both somewhat tormented by the ways we're conventional and the ways we go against the grain. But it's my daddy who made me a writer. When I was growing up, he would recite *The Love Song of J. Alfred Prufrock* and *Kubla Khan* on road trips, two poems that have become all-time favorites of mine, not surpassed by even Ginsberg's *Howl* in my Naropa days. And on childhood winter nights, at that big wooden dinner table surrounded by windows in the eating area off our kitchen, he would recite Robert Frost's *Fire and Ice.* Followed sometimes, after dinner by the fire, with emotionally fierce renditions of Dylan Thomas's *Do Not Go Gentle Into That Good Night.* His eyes would well up. I didn't quite understand, as a kid, what it meant to not go gentle into a good night. But I'm thinking about that passion in his voice, and how I inherited it, during my great send-off to San Francisco.

My parents and Tor got out of bed to see me off. I hate good-byes; I especially hate saying good-bye to Tor. Leaving my sister breaks my heart, but I think what's hardest is that I'm leaving alone. And heading to a place where I will be alone: I don't have friends or family in San Francisco! My friends and family are in Virginia! Right here in this driveway as I back out slowly and wave, breathing deeply into the Virginia dawn and hitting the road solo.

I set out on Interstate 64, having just turned twenty-five and newly out of credit card debt, thanks to a last-minute yard sale and parental donation. The Jetta my dad bought me is packed with as much as I could fit (including a down comforter and several boxes of books).

This move to California is a courageous step for me. Over the next three and a half days, I drive the entire width of the United States of America, from Virginia to California. I take a late-night phone call from Aaron (who I miss sorely) in a hotel room near the middle of the country. I drive right past the signs for Boulder when I switch directions at Denver and head north, into Wyoming. I whoop it up through Nevada, screaming *Holy hell!* and jacked on caffeine, crying and spitting and drawing on my thigh, skirt pulled up high, shaking my hair, screaming as loud as I can, losing my voice. I feel the liberation of the open road, the freedom of being young and unattached, and the thrill of my adventures before me. This is a sweet, rich, and beautiful experience.

But I also pull into a hotel by 5:30 P.M. every evening to make sure it isn't dark when I check in alone. I find a gym in each location so I can run a few miles on the treadmill before finding some cheap, fast-food dinner. I call my parents often, and I sleep hardly at all, waking up before dawn and hitting the road again each morning. The experience takes only a few days, but it's truly epic.

When I finally roll into San Francisco, I'm equipped with a map and a key to an apartment; a friend of Charlotte's is generous enough to let me stay at her place in Nob Hill while she's out of town. I almost wreck my car driving on the steep San Francisco grades—we have hills in Virginia, but this is *crazy!*

Eventually, I make it. Not only to my temporary home, but into a more permanent one, a small apartment in the Castro that I share with another girl in my MFA program.

I headed off to San Francisco feeling just about fully recovered. I had relapsed in Virginia. I had learned many a thing the hard way. I know that big changes are hard for me—prone to anxiety and starvation—but I feel more capable than ever of tackling this exciting new venture.

And I'm right to be confident. I'm right to go. I am recovered. Because I know by now that recovery doesn't mean an A+ report card 100% of the time. Recovery means knowing how to act quickly, to respond to the negative pulls of an eating disorder swiftly enough to prevent dangerous relapse. And I know that I'll have many occasions to draw on these skills in my new San Francisco life. I make a couple of friends who are obsessed with their bodies and what they eat. I have to constantly tell myself that I am *me* and I do not need to compare my body to theirs. Plus, school is challenging—so many new changes, so much to get used to. A part of me wants to rely on food for comfort, and I'm beginning to recognize this, so I hire a dietitian. And then I hire a therapist.

It's not that I'm in any dangerous position. What I'm doing is simple: recognizing my potential for relapse. Recognizing how scared I am by some of the new challenges in my life and taking preventative action to keep myself on track. I meet with my dietitian for only a couple of months, as food isn't really that much of an issue. But I stay with my therapist for over two years, always finding value in an hour a week to work on being stronger, learning to cope with every crossroads with a bit more confidence.

I am dating a Stanford PhD candidate named Wallace who doesn't understand at first why I need therapy. My weight is healthy; I am eating flexibly, exercising moderately and regularly, not exhibiting signs of serious depression or anxiety. But when I explain to Wallace the potential I feel inside me, the fear of going back to where I'd once been, and the fierce, loving voices of my first dietitian, Anne, and my favorite therapist, Samuel, I know that choosing to get help before a problem escalates can never be a mistake.

And I do have a few bad moments: one or two nights of panic that lead to bingeing followed by intense cardio sessions at the gym, one insane day of trying to sustain myself on fruit because I hadn't had a bowel movement in several days, and a few nights of sleeplessness. Relapse is real when dealing with eating disorders. Someone who once found solace in overexercising or undereating is never going to forget the sense of (false) calm she gleaned from those controlling behaviors. But once you've gone through treatment, you'll never forget the joy and freedom you feel from really living. I know my self-abusing past did not offer any lasting security. I know the only way to find that truly is to trudge slowly forward through the muck and skate gleefully on sunny days.

# FALL 2005

After a year of city life, I move into a small apartment in Palo Alto, about forty-five minutes south of San Francisco. I've become familiar with the town, famous for being the home of Stanford University, through dating Wallace, and even though our yearlong relationship is deteriorating fast and I know it, I still want to escape to the suburbs.

In Palo Alto I begin to build my business. I'm personal training again, like I did in Virginia, going to people's homes and helping women develop exercise plans that are sensible, pleasurable, and right for them. But in Palo Alto I have more clients. I have more clients, more confidence; people listen to me, stay with me, rely on me. Plus, it's bigger here. Better pay, better results. I've learned a lot about relating to people, about myself, about supporting someone else while still managing to take care of myself. Life out west is good.

Wallace and I break up about a week after I move to Palo Alto, and I get over it quickly. I'm deeply engaged in the second and final year of my MFA and working on a French translation project. I'm studying the language with a private tutor, translating Rimbaud, and working on my thesis: an original manuscript of my own poems. I start a book club in Palo Alto, where I make friends with several smart and sassy women who challenge and inspire me. I'm also taking private tennis lessons and swimming a few days a week at the YMCA.

I've lived in so many fabulous towns by this point in my life: first and foremost Charlottesville, the most subtly gracious and elegant town I've ever known, but also Boulder, Boston, San Francisco, and now Palo Alto. Paly is different. It's California suburban chic, with plenty of strip malls: these brand-new, less-than-charming rectangular stucco buildings that happen to house fabulous restaurants. I feel safe in Palo Alto. I love my clients here, I love my private tennis and French lessons, I love my new girlfriends, and I love the YMCA. And the public library. And the smell of eucalyptus trees everywhere.

I'm happy, I'm confident, I'm working under the tutelage of brilliant poets, and I'm single. So I get on match.com and start lining up dates.

# JANUARY 25, 2006

Jeffrey and I have our first date at a British pub in Menlo Park, a town northwest of Palo Alto. I'm frantic when I arrive: My thesis is due in May, and my computer crashed last night. I've just spent all day at the Apple store in downtown Palo Alto trying to reckon with the "geniuses" there, but I wind up buying a brand-new laptop and having to type everything in again from the hard copies I luckily have.

Slowly I start to unwind: Jeffrey and I drink beer and talk about skiing, NPR (we have the same favorite show: *Fresh Air* with Terry Gross!), and Boston. He lived there, too, for a while. But he's originally from California, even though he looks like a preppy East Coaster who belongs on a rainy Main Street somewhere. He's four or five years older than me and the handsomest man I've ever been on a date with, hands down. He has a perfectly shaped face: not pretty-boy chiseled, but balanced features, with warm eyes and a full head of hair, clean cut. He's a landscape architect with better manners than any Virginian, and he's quiet at first.

After two dates he takes a job in Sacramento, a traffic-filled two- or three-hour drive from Palo Alto, and I think I'll never see him again. But then he starts inviting me to ski in Tahoe practically every weekend, and before I know it, I'm splitting my time between Palo Alto and Sacramento and building a relationship with a brilliant new boyfriend who makes me feel like a bright and beautiful woman.

# July 12, 2006

I've just left Jeffrey's apartment, and I'm driving west on I–80, home to Palo Alto from Sacramento.

It's July. It's hot in California, especially in the valley; temperatures are breaking records at well over 100 degrees, and I'm grateful for a car with excellent air-conditioning and the decaf iced Americano I picked up from Starbucks before I started my drive. It's too hot for the jeans I'm wearing, and my bra is rubbing uncomfortably under my arm. The phone has been ringing too much lately. I'm tired of talking to people. I'm blasting the radio, but somehow I still hear the ring of my cell beneath the music.

It's been an exciting season for me. In May I graduated from California College of the Arts with my MFA in creative writing, and my parents and brother flew out to hear my final reading. Plus, a four-page spread all about me appeared in *People* magazine. I was interviewed about my recovery and my work now as a trainer, and it snowballed into a series of media appearances and interviews, including a chance to appear live on *The View* and meet Barbara Walters. My mom came with me, and we giggled in our New York hotel room over graham crackers and peanut butter.

The five minutes of fame has been fun, but I'm enjoying Jeffrey more. Sacramento is becoming a second home to me, despite its cow-town reputation for being San Francisco's ugly stepsister. I kinda like it, though: less pretentious than Paly, cute old homes, and of course, the best boyfriend of all time.

Jeffrey and I have just taken a long weekend to hike Mt. Whitney, the tallest mountain in the continental U.S., and

I'm telling this to the man who is now interviewing me over the phone. He's writing an article for a small Virginia paper about exercise addiction, and he wants to know how it makes me feel now when I see women working out as hard as I used to. Dry, golden reeds of grass are flying behind me as I drive. I'm speeding. Everyone speeds in California. I'm learning to respond to interviewers' questions without really answering them, like how politicians manage to get their message across regardless of what they're asked. But this question I take time to answer, though I answer it indirectly.

When I was sick, when I was underweight, when I had made my world so small, when all that mattered was how little I ate and how far I ran, when I lived in my mom's little white apartment on Little High Street in Charlottesville, I couldn't remember life before my disorder. I didn't know it was a disorder; it was a passion. I stood one day in the bathroom at the top of the stairs in Mom's tidy apartment and I looked at my narrow, white face in the mirror and I touched my bony cheeks. I had just been flipping through photographs from my life with Christopher, photographs of me and Christopher on a short hike from the car to the coast in Oregon that summer of our Pacific road trip, in 2000. We took turns mooning the camera, and my hair was so long and unbrushed, and I was wearing Christopher's sweater and an old pair of jeans. And my ass. Coming out of my pants. And Christopher's out of his, and it made me shy to look at those pictures. So I stood in front of the mirror that day in Mommy's apartment, several years ago now, and I touched my cheek and I thought, *Really? I did that? I really did that? What does it feel like to kiss a man?* I couldn't remember. I couldn't remember the feeling; I couldn't conjure the sensation, lip on lip, tongue on tongue, tongue on skin, skin on skin, skin on lip. I was sexless, so far removed from a life of pleasure and feeling. I didn't recognize the girl with her juicy ass coming out of her dirty jeans. I didn't recognize the girl who would do that for her boyfriend's camera. I didn't recognize the girl who had a boyfriend.

Now, driving home from Sacramento, I'm thinking about the sex Jeffrey and I had the other night in a hotel room on our drive back through the Sierras, home from Mt. Whitney. We watched ourselves in the big hotel mirrors. He held my body with his hands and we kissed passionately, craning our necks to watch our bodies moving in the mirror. We had just come from dinner in a steak house in the town of Mammoth, and I'd had a little wine, so my cheeks were flushed and my body gently pulsing. This Peach couldn't get enough of her naked body, together with Jeffrey's, in the mirror.

And that Peach—the woman who was half drunk and making love with her boyfriend—that's the same spirit of the girl who mooned Christopher's camera hiking in Oregon. That's the same girl I didn't recognize in that sad, shiny mirror on Little High Street. And that night, with Jeffrey in the mirrors in Mammoth, I could not recognize the Peach who was skinny, sick, and desperate to run.

When I stop for traffic on my hot drive back to Palo Alto, head twisted to the side to hold the cell phone in place while I'm on the line with the interviewer from Virginia, I take a second to look in the mirror at my full, radiant cheeks, and I touch them. I can feel Jeffrey's hands on my body and his lips on my face. I can bring back the other night in Mammoth, but

I can't feel, I can't bring back, I can't conjure the sunken white face of the girl who didn't eat, the girl who ran too far, the girl who wouldn't stop running until she'd injured joints in every corner of her body and couldn't walk up the stairs.

*I don't relate anymore,* I tell the man on the phone. I know that I did that, starved myself and ran too far, I have pictures, I talk and write about it, but I don't recognize that version of myself anymore. I don't feel her in me, and I don't know how I did it. I just climbed a mountain this past weekend, and I'm tired, and I can't wait to take the next few days off to eat and watch movies and sleep.

And all that's true: how far removed I feel. But what's also true is the knowledge that I did run my body into the ground, and I could do it again. Even this recovered, even hardly recognizing my sick, skinny self, I know somehow, intellectually, that if I wanted to, some part of me could still carve out shapes from every inch of arm and leg, from every cell of stomach and thigh. I could waste away and never come back and stare into mirrors and remember sex and kissing without really being able to remember it. I know that that potential is in me, somewhere, buried beneath all the hard work I've done to return to my zesty, happy self. I could, but I don't ever want to. I'm programmed differently now. I'm programmed with years of therapy, with enough skills and tools that even on autopilot I answer back at my compulsive side with automatic nos. Now I can only go forward. And driving through a hot California summer, on a shimmering freeway stacked so steadily with cars I can hardly see through them to read the road signs, I'm happy to be driving to my Palo Alto apartment where I can see my Palo

Alto friends and readily conjure my weekend: the sensation of gritty sex in a tent, the sensation of sweat against my backpack, the exhilaration of standing on the summit of Mt. Whitney with my California boyfriend in the gleaming California sun.

I hang up with the interviewer, sip my iced coffee, and zip toward Paly, shades on, nodding my head along with the radio.

# JULY 21, 2006

We always say, *It used to be that you knew everybody on these tiny propeller planes into Charlottesville,* but the last time I said it, I realized I couldn't actually remember a time when that was true. Today I know nobody flying into Charlottesville. Okay, one man looks familiar, but I decide it's just that he's pretty and looks like he lives on a horse farm, so I probably don't know him, just his archetype.

I'm thinking horribly cruel thoughts about the awkward, plain-looking stewardess whose smile seems to be held in place by fear. I'm connecting in Cincinnati, heading to Charlottesville for a short weekend in Virginia for my childhood friend Kristen's wedding. Kristen and I don't keep up with each other's lives that much anymore, but I still love her dearly and can't wait to watch her get married. Anyway, I'm trying to discern whether this stewardess (we're supposed to say *flight attendant* now?) is Charlottesville- or Cincinnati-based. I silently hope Cincinnati, but honestly it could go either way. The case in point here is that Charlottesville has grown since I was a little girl—not only do I not recognize the individual people on the plane with me, but I don't know how to identify the type of person each of them is. And how they fit into the Charlottesville stereotypes I've long understood.

My parents pick me up Friday evening. I love landing in Charlottesville in the summer. I love looking out the window and slowly descending on the rolling green hills. I love how small and womanly the mountains are. They don't reach up begging, dangerously teetering on an edge like the mountains out west do—instead, they slowly rise, politely, delicately, humbly, not asking to be noticed, really, but offering comfort to whatever lies below. They are still comforting from above, and as I begin to recognize the redbrick buildings and white columns of southern architecture coming into focus, I well up about being home.

Mom and Dad are standing in the little shop in the airport. They're talking to a grown daughter and her elderly mother—*I knew it!* The man I sort of recognized, I do know his family, and now I can place him: the grown daughter's brother. I guess Charlottesville hasn't changed as much as I thought.

At the wedding on Saturday it's old Charlottesville: familiar faces everywhere, everyone understood, perfectly categorized, properly playing out their roles in a comforting and sort of terrifying way. Earlier, before the wedding, we had lunch at Feast, and I saw three kids I went to high school with. No longer kids, of course: Shep and June are married and were toting their baby around (I hadn't heard!), and Cinder looked just like her mother. I felt immediately shy. I regress in Charlottesville; I'd put on my little sister's dress to wear that day and looked like a teenybopper slut, sort of, with my boobs falling out and my hair in my face. What I like about Charlottesville is my total ease in the town. It's the sort of place where I feel safe enough to wear a lacy push-up bra under a pink polka-dot dress that's low cut enough to show half the bra, and to top it all off with a big floppy straw hat. And I actually think it looks good—that is, until I bump into peers from high school who were just older enough and just cooler enough that I want to cling to my parents and pretend I don't see them.

Later, at the wedding, I stand next to Cinder for a photo with our arms around each other. Then we talk like we are old friends, and a part of me wishes we could be. All the high school trivialities that used to come between us are gone, like I knew they would be. Leaving the restaurant at lunch, Dad asked, *Why didn't you say hi?* And I said, *Oh, you know, this is how we do it—pretend we don't see each other and then act like best friends at the wedding tonight.* I don't have a lot of logic to explain that; it's just part of the Charlottesville etiquette. Or non-etiquette, or lingering immaturity, or status and hierarchy obsession that half of us can't quite grow out of.

Several people at the wedding say to me, *You look great,* and one old friend says, *You look better than ever,* and I know people are responding to how I looked in the throes of my disorder. It's Beatrice, a girl I knew peripherally for most of my life, who tells me I look better than ever, and it feels sincere and I'm so happy to see her and her sister Holly, who I was closer to though we had since lost touch. They look beautiful, too, with their husbands in the shedding light of dusk, and I want so badly, in that moment, to live back in Charlottesville with them, to marry one of their friends, to always go to weddings together at the country club and laugh about what we were like at seventeen and raise our babies together.

The sun drops. Everything is a numbing buzz: laughter, children, scuffing feet and soft music, the clinking sound of glasses. Me. I'm standing just outside that big white tent. Watching my beautiful old friends dance with their husbands, their fathers, and then I'm dancing with my father, laughing, loving him with my biggest, most open and least judgmental heart. Right now I want nothing more than to find a way to be the perfect Charlottesville woman. Watching Kristen and her new husband cut the cake, I can't stop crying so I turn to my mother and say, *I'm so jealous,* which is true, but I'm also deeply moved by the love between a man and a woman and their willingness to commit so unabashedly to spending their lives together, faithfully. And to myself I say, *I am staring everything in the face that I don't have and didn't think I wanted, but suddenly do.*

Which doesn't mean that I didn't think I wanted marriage and love. I have always wanted marriage and love. But I didn't think I wanted it in a country club. I didn't think I wanted the sense of belonging to this community that suddenly I feel desperate for. And then I realize, wait, I do belong to this community. I am here. Everyone I see is hugging me. Everyone is asking about my life. E-mail addresses are being exchanged. This is a world that will always be mine, that can't disappear, that I don't have to cling to, hold onto, in order to always be a part of. In fact, no matter what I do this town is in my blood and bones and I'm stuck with it. With everyone who knew me in elementary school and everyone they're now married to. And I'm blissfully happy about this fact.

I fly back to California on Sunday. And when my plane lands I'm anxious, I'm anxious for it to get on the ground, just to put the weekend behind me, to see Jeffrey and to clean my apartment and to resolidify *my* life, the one that I made for myself by choice, not the one I was born into. I go to the grocery store, I leave messages for half my friends, I take a nap and jog near the path by the park, I condition my hair and change my sheets. Mine. California. Mine.

# MAY 19, 2007

Jeffrey proposes to me huddled over a Whisperlite camp stove at Helen Lake on Mt. Shasta. It's nearly dusk.

One morning during the first winter when we were dating, I was shuffling around Jeffrey's bedroom, tugging my boots on over my jeans and throwing my favorite green and blue knee-length sweater across my shoulders, when I looked up and caught Jeffrey sitting up in bed, head cocked to the side, staring at me with this look of clarity in his smile. Now, you have to take my word for it, but Jeffrey has the most incredible smile known to man. I'm biased, admittedly, but it's true that he is blessed with a pair of deep eyes like those sweet Virginia lakes, eyes that well with sensitivity and when paired with a genuine tooth-smile, reveal a fall-flat-on-your-face sexy beckoning that burns me to my core. In that moment, though, he wasn't coming on to me, he was just . . . looking.

*What?* I asked. He straightened out his head and said to me, deadpan, *You're, like, a normal, well-adjusted girl. You don't have any hang-ups or anything. I like you. Ha!* I thought to myself and only told Jeffrey months later, *I can't wait to tell my old therapists you said that!*

Now we're on a snowy mountain in May, a season when most people are ready to embrace tank tops and sunny beaches. But this is California, remember, and we have any season we want at any time of year. Mt. Shasta is snowy. Period. We have been hiking all day, with full packs, up to Helen Lake, which is not really a lake but an area where the mountain levels off at over 10,000 feet. Jeffrey has run off to melt snow, and he's been gone for over an hour. I finish setting up camp and then perch by our tent, bundled up, gazing at the view: snowcapped peaks in the distance, and down below, the little yellow glittering lights of the town of Mt. Shasta beginning to stand out as the sun slowly sets. I am brutally exhausted. This mountain is a beast. We have tried hiking it twice before and made it once nearly (oh so very nearly) to the summit, but I backed down that time, fear and fatigue getting the better of me at the bottom of Misery Hill, Shasta's home stretch. We backpacked farther up today, thinking this will help us reach the summit tomorrow morning, but now I'm feeling like carrying the weight of my pack those extra miles is only going to help me sleep in tomorrow and forget the summit altogether. (As it turns out, that's what happens, but not necessarily because we were tired. As it turns out, the purpose of this trip had little to do with mountain climbing; it had to do with *marriage*.)

Jeffrey finally returns from melting snow, and we set up the stove to cook dinner. We're making soup from a dried mix, and it isn't cooking fast enough for my growling belly. To pass the time I say, *Hey, honey, tell me a story. No, tell me a secret!* He looks at me for a second and says, *Really? Okay* . . . and then reaches into his pocket.

Time does stop—this is not a dramatization. Time stops, and I can't actually experience the moment because I'm pretty sure I leave my body. Jeffrey is asking me to marry him. And I burst into tears. He is crying, too, though without those emotional (and loud!) heaves and sniffles, and he tells me that he called my daddy yesterday to get his blessing. He has just revealed this gorgeous diamond and sapphire ring, and I'm thinking, *Wow, you hiked all the way up here with that!? What if you'd lost it!?* But all I can do is cry and cry and then I realize I need to say something and I grab his cold, windblown face and kiss it and say, of course, *Yes!* We kiss some more. We pet each other. We hug and our faces are snotty and cold and my tears are running into my scarf and after a few minutes a group of nearby climbers applauds.

I don't sleep all night. For one, the wind is so fierce our tent poles are literally bending in, reaching nearly to our noses. I cuddle up to Jeffrey, who sleeps a little but not much, and he tells me everything is going to be okay, it's just windy. To me, this is dangerous. To me, this is a bad situation. But my now fiancé is steady as ever and shhhhs me to sleep. Though I never quite make it. I dig around for my headlamp, switch it on, and stare at my new ring. I'm getting married. I'm getting married. I'm getting married.

In the morning we sleep in and hike out. Who needs to climb a mountain? We're getting married! I wear the ring under my gloves for the hike down and giddily describe it to Tor, who is the first person I call, as promised (a pact of sisterhood: You are the first to share news about sex, engagements, and probably pregnancy, but we're not there yet), when we get back to our car and park in the town of Mt. Shasta. Next I call my mother, who cries into the phone. My entire family of course already knew, since Jeffrey had called Daddy the day before. My brother Nat even gets weepy on the phone. When I reach him he's in the airport, heading back to Munich, where he lives now with his German girlfriend. After I finish my emotional family phone calls, Jeffrey takes me for eggs and coffee at our favorite breakfast spot in Mt. Shasta. Walking on air.

I wasn't sick with my eating disorder for a decade, like many women are (many, in fact, suffer for an entire lifetime).

But I was sick enough and for long enough to recognize, in joyous moments in life such as this, that living a full life is a most remarkable experience. There were days during my illness and recovery that I wondered if I'd ever lead a normal, functioning life again. I remember once having a conversation with my mother about whether I would live my whole adult life at home, under her care. When I was deep in that black hole of compulsive exercise, starvation, and depression, I could not have imagined living in California, climbing Mt. Shasta, and eating eggs with my fiancé. *Fiancé!* Life is good indeed.

# Epilogue

*Every Sunday morning as a little girl, I'd wake up to the smell of Mom's French pancakes cooking on the griddle. They weren't like the pancakes I'd have at my friends' houses when I spent the night: fluffy and made with buttermilk, where the imitation syrup would soak through and make the cake all soggy. These were different: flat, dense, and perfect, glazed with butter and real maple syrup. They were a thicker version of a crepe. I'm making them now, for Jeffrey, wondering every time I do this if they'll ever be as good as Mom's. And there's no exact science, because Mom never measured. Thus, I inherited all our favorite meals sans grams or cups. To Mom it's all about* eyeballing *or* feeling it out.

*I usually make a test pancake and then adjust the batter. This time the test comes out too thin, so I add flour and a little oil. The rest come out perfectly; the brown maplike pattern from the butter on the skillet imprinted on each side of the cake gives a paper-thin layer of crusty texture. Butter slides off the pile of pancakes and onto the plate. I put chocolate chips in two or three of them, like Mom did some Sundays, when I begged her enough or when she was happy enough. We sit at the table together, Jeffrey and I, in our new apartment in Sacramento, and wash them down with orange juice.*

## A Difference in Motivation

I still work out regularly. During a recent interview a woman asked me, *What's the difference?* I explained the key difference: motivation. When I was an exercise bulimic, I was motivated by a desire to purge. I felt somehow wrong for eating. I felt fat. I felt full and that made me hate myself. I ran, I swam, I danced, I lifted, I did all of this to get rid of something—of myself. These days, I work out five or six days a week for about an hour, sometimes more, sometimes less. But when I'm sick, I rest. And when I don't feel like it, I don't exercise. And when I go on vacation, I chill out and enjoy myself. I'm flexible about the time of day I hit the gym or the road, and I'm flexible, too, about what sort of exercise I'm getting. In fact, the more variety, the better: I ski, I run, I play tennis, I hike, I swim, I lift, I practice yoga, I walk, I dance, and I'll try anything new.

I'm motivated by many things, now, but nowhere in my motivation is a need to purge. My friends, my fiancé, my family—I still appreciate their occasional concern. I am glad, grateful that they stop sometimes to say, *Are you sure you need to go running today?* Or *Why don't you take a day off?* I'm glad also that I can answer them with the confidence that I'm in it for the right reasons. Among my list of motivators are to care for my health, to be a better trainer for my clients, to enjoy the outdoors, to be social, to challenge myself, to try new things, to change my mood, to breathe deeply.

It took me several years of deliberate, conscious work to be able to use exercise as a positive tool in my life. I used to confuse, for instance, taking care of my health with losing weight. Now when I think about taking care of my health, I think about preventing osteoporosis and heart disease. I think about de-stressing: taking in deep breaths, relaxing, having some time to clear my head. I also remember everything I learned in my personal trainer classes, which included the risks of overtraining. In order to care for my health, I can't overdo it. I cross-train now to avoid injury. I get extra sleep on days when I work out a lot (e.g., when I have to exercise with clients), and I keep myself fueled throughout the day. I drink lots of water, and I eat often.

## Avoiding Triggers

My relationship with running, specifically, has changed. Running is a popular sport for compulsive exercisers: It's addictive, it's efficient, and it's accessible. I do not generally recommend that an exercise bulimic who was a runner pick that sport up again until she feels solidly recovered. Any practice that was a part of someone's addiction can trigger that person back into that behavior. An ex-smoker who used to have a cigarette every time he or she went out for drinks with friends, for example, is encouraged to stop drinking as well.

It took me years to feel like I could run for the right reasons again. Now that I'm in a healthy, respectful relationship with my body and exercise, I can enjoy the feeling of a good road run. I love the rhythm, the air in my face, the feeling of sweat building under my skin. But because of my knee problems and my history with using running as a means to purge, today I keep my runs short. I keep them short and infrequent, and this is how I manage that relationship.

When I go to the pool to swim, I follow a plan that Jeffrey, who was a star swimmer when he was in school, writes for me. When I go to a yoga class, I'm conscious of my history of shoulder injuries, and I take opportunities to rest in child's pose. And when I go to the gym to lift, I emulate the plans that I write for my own clients. The rest of the time I'm with friends, playing tennis or skiing, hiking or taking walks around town, and this is my favorite way to exercise now. With all of these tools in my back pocket, I'm taking action every day to care for myself and to prevent a relapse.

Staying recovered from my eating disorder is no longer a daily battle. I no longer have to fight it, reckon with it, or even talk to it like I did in the early days of recovery. But in some sense, I am always in a degree of dialogue with that part of my past, because recovery isn't about achieving perfection; it's about developing the confidence to create a life that keeps me healthy and whole, about learning to care for myself in a way that prevents relapse and that lets me function day to day healthfully, happily, and able to give back.

## Perspective and Identity

A friend in recovery recently e-mailed to ask me how I learned to accept my body size post–eating disorder. Before I wrote her back, I thought for a minute about how to respond, and two key words came to mind: perspective and identity.

I don't have a clear-cut answer to the question *How did you recover, Peach?* I sometimes wish I did, though, especially when parents ask me for help with their daughters or sons, or when those struggling through treatment are looking for inspiration themselves. Everyone wants that secret remedy, a potion they can take before bed at night to wake up refreshed, happy, and healthy; unfortunately, the reality is an average of three to seven years of treatment. It can be grueling, but it's also an opportunity that most people never have: to step away from day-to-day tasks and take time with trained professionals who are there to help you look deep inside yourself and get to know who you are beneath the neurosis. In this way, treatment is a luxury. In no way do I mean to diminish the challenges of treatment: they are innumerable and sometimes unbearable. Still, in many ways I see myself as fortunate for having gone through my eating disorder, and especially through treatment and recovery. I have a sense of myself, of who I am, what I want, and what I believe in, that I never would have achieved without treatment.

For me it was one initial leap of faith followed by lots of trial and error: false starts, setbacks, confused, crying nights and occasional blissful intervals that ultimately lead me forward, away from the disease and into myself. Recovery does not happen in an instant. But if for one moment we can be convinced that it might be worth fighting for, well, that moment can multiply into many moments (albeit often shadowed by doubt and intermingled with self-loathing and confusion) that slowly but eventually become the majority of moments. It felt like an eternity when I was inching my way through recovery, but now, looking back, I see why it took time. We cannot change ourselves overnight. Habits that have developed over years cannot be unlearned immediately.

It went kind of like this: I would have a mini-epiphany or a feeling of pure fear, like when Anne told me, *You're going to die if you don't stop this*—some sort of realization that motivated me to try something new, to make a change, to put some effort into recovery. And then I'd take a risk, trust my doctors, and, for example, take a day off running. I'd get through the day, somehow, and look back to see that not much had changed. I was still here on this planet, I was still about the same size, my friends and family were still around me somewhere, and no major catastrophe had ensued.

That doesn't mean I didn't cry and toil over it—I did, absolutely. But I proved to myself, in baby steps, that change wasn't really *so* terrible. Of course, after so many of these baby steps had accumulated, real changes had been made, and that was terrifying. But again I could check myself and say, *I'm still here. I'm still here, I'm breathing, I'm okay.* I couldn't really say any longer, *I'm still about the same size,* because obviously, and thank goodness, I was gaining weight. But I could be at that slightly (and then later, significantly) larger size and see that I was still Peach. Undergoing major transformation, but again, still here, still breathing. Life could not have become much worse than one hundred pounds and ten-mile daily runs with no one to talk to and no laughter. Once I slowly began to recognize that, I realized that I had nowhere to go but up, even if the ride was going to be uncomfortable.

Growing up in a town like Charlottesville, in a wealthy, white community, I was surrounded by beautiful, thin women. A lot of attention was placed on money and style, and thinness often accompanies both. When I go back home to visit, I see it again: how my absolutely healthy and lean body is actually on the bigger end of the spectrum compared to the bodies of so many of the women I grew up with. Here, in my life in California, that just isn't so. I have friends who grew up, first of all, in a variety of socioeconomic classes. Not all of my friends grew up wealthy, and not all of my friends grew up with thin mothers. I have friends of different races and different body sizes. I am almost embarrassed to admit that I never had this diverse a peer group growing up.

I'm not trying to say that there's no pressure to be thin in California—indeed, this is the state that houses Hollywood, the state of celebrity madness and perpetual beach weather. Still, my community here is broad. And my client base is broad, too. Working as a personal fitness trainer, educating women to be healthy, to care for themselves from the inside out, has helped change my perspective. A significant part of my training clientele is sedentary or obese women who want to take better care of their health and simultaneously learn to accept their shape and size. I have so much love and compassion for them, and when I look at myself in the mirror with these women, I really, really love my body. Not because I am thinner than them, but because of how much appreciation and respect I have for their struggle. They remind me of where I've been, and that my body today is healthy, strong, and perfect in her own way.

I'm careful to observe my internal reactions to my clients, women who are sometimes morbidly obese and sometimes anorexic, and who would probably enjoy better health if they were to either lose or gain a significant amount of weight. At the end of the day, I feel inspired by my clients. I admire their struggle and the work they're doing to overcome it, which has helped shift my perspective about body size. It has also helped teach me about identity. I first began to explore this idea the fall of the year I moved to Boston. I wrote in my journal one September afternoon, *When suddenly you're no longer thin anymore, as a definition of who you are, you become actually yourself. When you don't have an outside to tie to your insides, you are forced to discover what your insides actually are, and then you are that, and no longer an anorexic.*

One reason that women have such a hard time recovering from eating disorders is that we base much of our identities in our bodies. At the gym recently I heard one woman ask another, *How was your weekend?* And the second woman responded, *Oh, my sister and I are doing the fat-free thing.* She didn't mention any activities or relationships beyond the fact that she and her sister were both resisting fat. When you have an eating disorder, the connections between you and your food, you and your workouts, and you and the voices of your disorder become the primary relationship. But personal relationships also play a significant role in the spectrum of illness and recovery.

When I broke up with Christopher, I was faced with the same sort of identity crisis that I was faced with again in my recovery. Without him, who am I? Without the roles that I play as his partner, what do I do? What choices do I make? And later, without my underweight body, who am I? Without my aggressive workouts, who am I? When Christopher and I broke up, I didn't know how to move forward in my life because my sense of identity had become enmeshed in my relationship. And after Christopher, my sense of identity became entangled in my eating disorder: tied to my weight, my workouts, my jeans size.

So how did I recover? By slowly unraveling my insides, so that I could begin to develop self-esteem, confidence, and identity founded in who I actually am, not what I've done or how I look. With these skills, I no longer needed to rely so heavily on the coping mechanisms of starvation and compulsive exercise. The more I learned to love myself (and oh, it was slow and sometimes ugly), the more my need to punish my body diminished.

An anorexic or bulimic often identifies a large percentage of her identity in her eating disorder or her body size. Usually, the younger the girl develops the eating disorder, the more difficult it is to recover, because she hasn't lived enough years to have an identity outside of that. I consider myself fortunate that I developed my eating disorder later, as a young adult. I had already lived through high school as a wild, spirited girl with an identity that had nothing to do with restriction, self-hatred, or thinness. In my recovery, this meant that I had previous experience to show me that there really is life outside of an eating disorder. I encourage my clients now to learn to identify outside their eating disorders and outside their bodies. It can help to look at your friends and family and learn to see their identities as separate from their sizes. If you make a list of what you love about your best friend or mother, it probably doesn't include her size or weight. Learning to see this same value in myself has helped me accept my natural body size. I am many things, and I'm housed in a body. It's useful.

Instead of developing an eating disorder, it would have been nice if I had known other ways of searching for answers, other ways to cope, so that I would not have had to experience so much pain or put my loved ones through so much pain. But I don't regret it. I don't regret it because, through the recovery that followed, I discovered a true sense of myself that I never had before. And now that I'm with the man I will live with until death do us part, I am grateful for the soul-searching journey that made me the woman I am today: healthy, aware, and a whole lot less afraid. As I write this book and revisit moments in my past, I realize that I could not be the Peach of today, marrying Jeffrey, if I had not endured all that murk and muck. I would not be capable of loving Jeffrey the way that I am able to now. And this makes me deeply grateful for my journey.

## Cultural Influences and Eating Disorders

The leaders in America's health industry emphasize the need for regular exercise and attention to diet. Obesity is an epidemic, childhood obesity is on the rise, and new weight-loss programs appear every year. Shows like NBC's *The Biggest*

*Loser* gain mass attention, and every tabloid on the grocery store shelves showcases a celebrity who has recently lost, or gained, a noticeable amount of weight. We scrutinize ourselves, our role models, our friends and family. This obsession with food, fitness, and body image translates into a prevalence of eating disorders. Citing expert research, the National Eating Disorders Association estimates that up to 10 million women and 1 million men in America are currently battling some form of anorexia or bulimia and that another 25 million are struggling with binge eating disorders.

Anorexia has a dramatically high premature death rate in comparison to other mental illnesses, along with an unfortunately low recovery rate. And this subject matter is timelier than ever: New studies have identified a genetic component in the development of anorexia nervosa. My story is consistent with this evidence, as my mother battled a severe case of anorexia in her youth. Research for exercise bulimia is not as comprehensive, as it's still a relatively new eating disorder, and the terminology is less clear. Is it treated as bulimia? Is it treated as anorexia, since the two compulsions often occur together? Is it treated as an eating disorder or as an exercise disorder?

I view exercise bulimia as an eating disorder because the behavior stems from a desire to purge calories. To an exercise bulimic, the point of working out is to relieve the guilt associated with eating. The method differs from traditional bulimia, but the motive is much the same.

I explained to a new friend recently why an exercise compulsion is so dangerous. We were taking a walk together at a park in Sacramento on a bright California day. The sun was in my eyes, and I wished I'd worn a baseball cap. She was asking questions like, *But isn't it good to be addicted to exercise? I mean, we're taking a walk now because this is healthy, right? There's an obesity epidemic, it's a major problem with children—isn't it okay to be addicted to fitness?*

I'm much better than I used to be about responding to questions like these. *Actually,* I pointed out, *an exercise compulsion is extremely dangerous.* I explained that it's often coupled with anorexia and that it's life threatening. I offered the information that those who overexercise put themselves at risk for heart attack and heart failure, that they destroy their metabolisms. I also revealed some of the psychological qualities of an exercise addiction: isolating yourself from family and friends; prioritizing workouts over social functions, vacations, or holidays; and experiencing extreme anxiety and guilt when unable to exercise.

My friend wasn't wrong or even entirely misinformed to ask those questions. She's a typical American woman: concerned with her appearance and susceptible to the mass of information we're fed about how to care for our bodies. I understand this; I live it, too. Even now, in the grocery stores, Jeffrey steers me away from the magazine rack while we're waiting in line. *You're not supposed to look at those!* he chastises. He got this from me—I recently explained to him that when I was in treatment, I was encouraged to stay away from this sort of media influence until I was recovered enough to not be triggered by it. I told him that I usually wanted to be weighed facing away from the scale so that I couldn't read the numbers. I told him that my dietitian discouraged me from drinking diet soda or fat-free frozen yogurt. He took it all to heart, and it's nice. It's comforting to have someone love me and want me to stay well.

## Finding Balance—and Finding Yourself

I am well now, and reading magazines doesn't trigger me. I have learned to turn my compulsion with burning calories through exercise into a career. As a personal trainer, one who specializes in women's fitness, I make it my mission to educate clients properly on the risks of obsessive exercise. My perspective is unique in contemporary fitness: I do not focus on my clients' weight, measurements, or woes about their bodies. I focus instead on helping them learn to feel energized, strong, and capable, to develop a relationship with exercise that's about celebration and nourishment rather than punishment. Many women work out as a way of undoing. They work out to undo what they have eaten, to *lose* what they have gained. They are persuaded by magazines to *fix your tummy flaws* or *lose twenty pounds by summer,* and they develop a pattern of self-loathing that is perpetuated by our culture. My aim is to shift my clients' perspective to recognize that only through love, care, and nurturing can their bodies function well and can they feel good about themselves. I work with women who are overweight and underweight. I work with women who have perfectly healthy, balanced bodies. I work with menopausal women and adolescents. And the one thing these women all have in common when we first meet is some degree of hatred for their shape, some level of fear about who they are as a female body. Unfortunately, they are not alone. It is estimated that only 2% of women worldwide (*worldwide!*) describe themselves as beautiful. I'm on a mission to move these numbers up.

And numbers are a big part of the game. Exercise addicts are obsessed with counting in the same way anorexics are: They want to see calories burned go UP and calories consumed go

DOWN. They want to see their weight go DOWN, their time on a mile go DOWN, the total number of miles go UP. It's all about MORE and LESS and it's never enough. When my exercise bulimia was active, I would count steps in a run. I'd count one hundred steps on each of my ten fingers until I got to 1,000 and then start over. At some point I started to think of each step as a bite, and I focused on working off every bite I'd eaten with every step I ran. As an anorexic and bulimic, I felt a strong need to purge each and every one of the very few calories I allowed myself to eat. I was officially at war with my body. As soon as we track ourselves to fight our bodies, to fight our natural size and shape, like I did, we embark on a battle destined for failure. It is impossible to win when we fight who we are. We only move further from happiness, from health, and from freedom.

It's worth mentioning that an exercise addiction does not affect only those who are underweight and spending hours every day in the gym. A person can have an unhealthy, addictive obsession with exercise while still working out in moderate, recommended amounts. Some individuals may maintain a healthy body weight while exhibiting the psychological symptoms of an exercise compulsion, such as feeling the need to exercise on certain days at certain times in certain ways or, if that routine is not possible, feeling extreme guilt as a result.

## Recovery That Lasts

Of course, the long-term physical effects of exercise addiction can be devastating. In my own case, my joints have never fully recovered. I have more pain than my fifty-something-year-old mother, and some seasons I spend hours a week with ice on my knees or my shoulder. Even with moderate exercise, my body periodically revolts. This means I have to listen extra carefully and rest adequately, and when I start to feel pain, I have to back off—even if I'm not doing anything all that intense.

The other risks associated with exercise bulimia are similar to that of other eating disorders: The loss of the menstrual cycle, often associated with low-weight female athletes, can lead to osteoporosis early in life and to complications with fertility and/or pregnancy. When the body is at a low weight, the organs suffer. The heart can't function without adequate energy (calories) and will slow down to compensate. This is why heart failure is a risk with low-weight anorexia.

Many women *and* men (this illness is not exclusive to females) become addicted to exercise as a way of gaining control over their lives. It is true that obsessive, calculated workouts can help people feel a sense of security that they seek elsewhere in life and do not find. But as we know from observing a variety of addictions, this behavior becomes an escape from real life, and the sense of control is fleeting. An exercise addiction does not accomplish much in the way of developing a true, deep sense of security in the world. In fact, it sends people further away from such a state of being.

The issue of exercise bulimia is complicated by the drastic divide of eating disorders in contemporary culture (obesity as an epidemic vs. anorexic body-type fashion models), as well as the often-preached truth that we do, as humans, need to incorporate regular exercise into our lives as a way of staying healthy. Because obesity is a real concern today in America, we're bombarded by strategies and plans that tell us how much to exercise. Sometimes we're even told *the more the better.* Any women's magazine on the shelves today is shouting out two very clear messages: EAT LESS and EXERCISE MORE. These magazines are speaking to a population of people who are in some cases overweight and underexercised, but in other cases simply obsessed, dazzled, and confused (without knowing it) about what to put in their bodies and how to work it off.

The fact is, this topic sells. Women's magazines devote most of their pages to weight management because we'll pay to read about it. Between the diet industry and the fashion industry, we have starved our models and actresses while the weight of the average American woman continues to rise. I believe in cutting straight through both halves of this dangerous equation and educating women (and men!) to treat their bodies uniquely: Rather than assess their behaviors with the simplified charts in magazines, people should learn to listen to their own body signals, learn to treat themselves as valuable individuals, and let some of the voices that tell them they are too much of some things and not enough of others fall away.

This doesn't mean that there is never an appropriate time to hit the gym when you don't feel like it, or to make intentional choices to eat nutritious foods. But it means finding a way to do it that's first and foremost *right for you*. A way that has nothing to do with punishment, guilt, or fear. A way that is motivated by health and wellness. Above all, a way that is balanced. Working out obsessively is not balanced. Working out obsessively and starving yourself is not balanced. Working out obsessively and bingeing is not balanced. And never working out is not balanced.

I struggled for several years to understand what balance means in my own relationship to exercise and food. I slowly learned to define my body's desires and limitations, to develop a way of living happily in my body that keeps me energized and at peace with both food and fitness.

Recovering from any disorder or addiction is a process. When I'm interviewed, people often want clear answers about exactly when I got sick and exactly when I got better. I tell them it doesn't happen that way—recovery is two steps forward, one step back. Every step forward felt like I'd climbed a mountain, and sometimes I thought, *Now I'm here! Now I've done it!* before realizing that there was still work to do. Even now, as I educate professionally on the topic of compulsive exercise and eating disorders, my own work continues. As Jeffrey reminds me when he steers me from the magazines in Safeway, it's important that I continue to value my unique needs in order to ensure a recovery that lasts.

# Resources

National Eating Disorders Association (NEDA)
www.nationaleatingdisorders.org
Helpline: 800-931-2237
A not-for-profit organization, offering treatment referrals
and support for those suffering from anorexia, bulimia, binge
eating disorder, and individuals concerned with body image
and weight issues

Eating Disorder Referral and Information Center
www.edreferral.com
A comprehensive online listing of eating disorder treatment
providers all over the country

Something Fishy
www.somethingfishy.com
A listing of online chat rooms and support groups for people
suffering from eating disorders

Anorexia Nervosa and Related Eating Disorders, Inc.
(ANRED)
www.anred.com
A nonprofit organization that provides information about
eating disorders

# Acknowledgments

This book would not have been possible without the inspiration, support, and hard work of several important individuals to whom I am deeply grateful. I want to thank my editor, Lara Asher, for her insight and encouragement while refining this manuscript, and my agent Carol Mann for believing in it from the start. Thanks also to Imee Curiel, Laura Yorke, Mark Collins, and Margaret Kopp for their role in moving this manuscript forward, and to Joseph Lease, Donna de la Perriere, and Steffi Drewes for their belief in my work as a writer. Thanks to the incredible leaders at the National Eating Disorders Association, and my colleagues at Summit Eating Disorders and Outreach Program, for their mentorship, and for their dedication to such a worthy cause. Thanks to Steve Greenstein, Katherine Bruno, Anna Haupt, Whitney Moses, and Laura Pedersen for their love and patience through the worst of it. Heartfelt thanks to my brother, Nat, for believing in me when no one else did, and to my sister, Victoria, for her vibrant spirit and forgiveness. Thanks to my father for his willingness to let me grow, and to my mother for her fierce, unyielding support. Finally, thanks to my husband, Jeffrey Dumars, for walking into my world and taking me as I am.

# About the Author

**Peach Friedman** is a spokesperson for the National Eating Disorders Association (NEDA) and the Education and Outreach Coordinator for Summit Eating Disorders and Outreach Program. She is a personal fitness trainer who works with people recovering from eating disorders, and she has an MFA in creative writing. She has been featured in *People* magazine, has interviewed with Barbara Walters on ABC's *The View,* and has appeared on *20/20* and *E! True Hollywood Story.* She lives in Sacramento, California.